Atlas of Shoulder Surgery

Atlas of Shoulder Surgery

Richard J. Hawkins, M.D., FRCS(C)
Steadman Hawkins Clinic
Vail, Colorado

Robert H. Bell, M.D.
Orthopaedic Surgeons, Inc.
Akron, Ohio

Steven B. Lippitt, M.D.
Northeast Ohio Orthopaedic Associates, Inc.
Akron, Ohio

Illustrated by
Larry Howell
Steven B. Lippitt, M.D.

with 417 illustrations

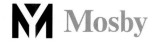 Mosby

St. Louis Baltimore Boston Carlsbad Chicago Naples New York Philadelphia Portland
London Madrid Mexico City Singapore Sydney Tokyo Toronto Wiesbaden

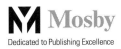

Mosby
Dedicated to Publishing Excellence

A Times Mirror
Company

Publisher: Anne Patterson
Editor: Robert Hurley
Developmental Editor: Lauranne Billus
Project Manager: Peggy Fagen
Designer: Judi Lang
Electronic Production Coordinator: Terri Bovay
Manufacturing Supervisor: Tony McAllister

Printed in the United States of America
Composition by Mosby Electronic Production
Printing/binding by The Maple–Vail Book Manufacturing Group

Mosby–Year Book, Inc.
11830 Westline Industrial Drive
St. Louis, Missouri 63146

International Standard Book Number ISBN 0-8151-4196-3

95 96 97 98 99 / 9 8 7 6 5 4 3 2 1

Special thanks to Barbara Dillman for her expert editorial skills in the final preparation of this manuscript and its illustrations.

Thanks to Dr. Robert Hancock of Athens, Georgia and Dr. Mark Dean of Beufort, South Carolina, both former fellows, who greatly aided in the final editing of the illustrations.

To our understanding families who support us in endeavors such as this *Atlas of Shoulder Surgery*.

Richard J. Hawkins
Robert H. Bell
Steven B. Lippitt

Preface

This book has been 7 years in the making and was motivated by the many visitors who come to us with a keen interest in spending time in the operating room and learning how to perform surgical procedures. Although important, surgery is only a part of the care of our patients. Nevertheless, attention to detail, careful technique, and an organized step-by-step approach can aid in maximizing the outcome. As surgeons, we take an appropriate history, perform a careful physical examination, and investigate where necessary to arrive at a diagnosis, but we have the privilege, through our surgery, to appreciate the pathology and the correction of that pathology as it relates to the patient's problem.

This *Atlas of Shoulder Surgery* was therefore written for those who wish to have a simple, practical, and illustrative approach to surgery of the shoulder. The set-up is such that on one page is a description of the operative procedure, and as closely aligned as possible, usually on the opposite page, is a plate of illustrations to detail that procedure. We have included almost all the operative procedures, whether common or unusual, that might be performed by an orthopaedic surgeon. In the description of the operation, we have offered a general discussion, provided the indications and contraindications, and elaborated on the surgical detail with carefully positioned illustrations. Finally, we have described the postoperative rehabilitation. Our goal was to keep the format simple, organized, and clear.

Shoulder surgery is a rapidly evolving field. We have included standard operations such as the classical Bankart reconstruction for anterior instability, and we have also described the newer procedures such as arthroscopic stabilization. We suspect in a few years' time, revision will be required to add still more procedures to this ever expanding field.

The most difficult challenge of such a text is to achieve the appropriate illstrations. We are indebted to Dr. Steven Lippitt, our co-author, a medical illustrator, a shoulder surgeon, and one who therefore understands anatomy and pathology of the shoulder. We are also indebted to his co-illustrator, Larry Howell, for finalizing these illustrations. It has been a monumental task for these two individuals to put all of this in place and make this text clear for our understanding of these operations. Rob Bell's experience and knowledge of shoulder surgery have aided greatly in the description of the operative procedures in this text.

This has been a project based on teamwork. It has been a labor of love. We hope that the readers of this book will understand the how-to of all these procedures. To you, the readers, enjoy! We hope that you learn and that you will find this text helpful in your understanding and application of shoulder surgery.

Richard J. Hawkins, M.D., FRCS(C)
Robert H. Bell, M.D.
Steven B. Lippitt, M.D.

Contents

Atlas of Shoulder Surgery

Introduction

This book shares our experiences with surgery for shoulder problems. The success of shoulder surgery lies only in part on the technical aspects and the operative procedure itself. The greater success is in an accurate diagnosis and careful judgment as to the surgical implications relating to that diagnosis. We follow certain protocols in operating room setup, positioning of the patient, instrumentation, and specifics of the surgical procedure.

Successful surgery depends on appropriate positioning of the patient on the operating table. (This positioning is described in the next chapter.) Successful surgery also depends on positioning of the arm, appropriate traction during certain phases of the surgery, and effective instrumentation for retraction. Retraction of various tissues, combined with traction and positioning of the arm, is critical to allow some degree of technical ease during surgery. Movement of the arm and specific positions will be described with each of the surgical procedures.

We have developed an instrumentation system for both a philosophical and a practical approach to retract structures in shoulder surgery. An open Bankart procedure is much easier with appropriate instrumentation. For example, use of a deltoid retractor and a pectoralis retractor, some form of anterior glenoid neck retractor to mobilize the Bankart lesion out of the way, and some form of humeral head retractor to pull the humeral head posteriorly while the Bankart repair is being performed all provide the means to effectively perform the repair. Different surgeons and companies have such retractors available that apply to certain procedures. The retractor system we developed is applicable to all shoulder surgery, including a self-retaining system (DePuy ProSource).

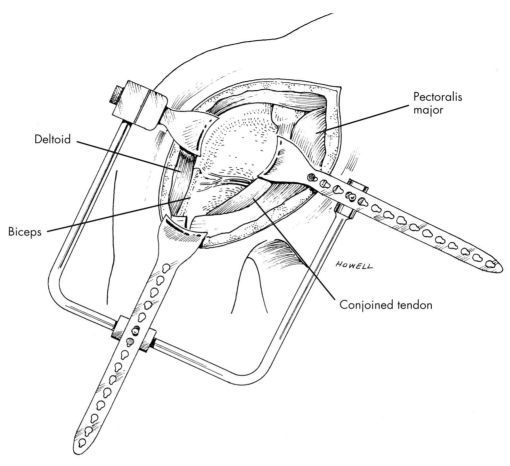

Deltoid

Biceps

Pectoralis
major

HOWELL

Conjoined tendon

FIGURE 1-1

The self-retaining system (Fig. 1-1) was developed especially for surgeons who have difficulty in obtaining assistance, for example, those in solo practice. The self-retaining instrument is designed to parallel the instrumentation we use for open procedures when there are adequate numbers of assistants. It is very effective for retracting to a certain depth, but once the capsular and interarticular tissues are reached, more specialized instruments that are not self-retaining are necessary.

General Approach to Surgical Procedures

We operate using a scalene block as often as possible. We often add a light general anesthetic if needed. The general approach to most surgical procedures follows a set pattern. The initial skin incision is taken through the subcutaneous level to the first muscular layer. At this time, self-retaining retractors are immediately positioned to create hemostasis by applying appropriate tension on the tissue and allowing easy visualization of the underlying structures. Fig. 1-2 shows self-retaining retractors and a modified Gelpi retractor exposing the underlying deltoid and cephalic vein in a routine deltopectoral approach. This procedure avoids the need to spend time controlling bleeding for hemostasis. Once the deeper levels are reached and these retractors are moved, bleeding is usually controlled.

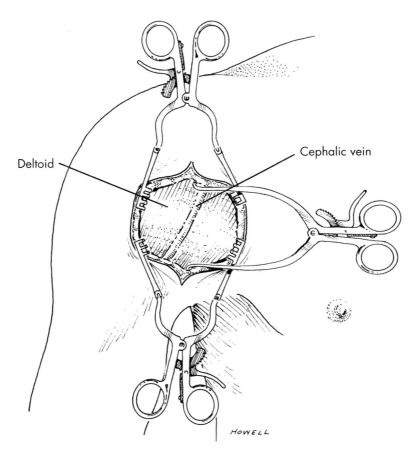

Deltoid

Cephalic vein

HOWELL

FIGURE 1-2

The next step in our approach is to appropriately retract the muscle layers out of the way. Initially, this can be done with various forms of right-angle retractors (Fig. 1-3). Similarly, when muscles are being mobilized out of the way, the self-retaining system is very applicable if assistance is unavailable. Fig. 1-1 shows the self-retaining system in place. It is mobilizing the deltoid laterally and the short flexors off the coracoid and pectoralis medially. It has an added retractor inferiorly to allow retraction inferiorly with an extended deltopectoral approach, as might be necessary in a total shoulder arthroplasty. This step exposes the underlying structures, such as the subscapularis, biceps tendon, and pectoralis raphe.

The next instruments from the set that are helpful depend upon the surgical procedure. If it is a rotator cuff repair or acromioplasty, we would mobilize the deltoid and place a retractor under the acromion to push the humeral head down. For example, in performing an anterior acromioplasty, this procedure allows exposure of the undersurface of the acromion (Fig. 1-4).

If we must proceed deeper through the anterior structures of the shoulder, we then retract the deltoid. We use the deltoid retractor that goes under the acromion, under the deltoid, and over the rotator cuff. This allows one finger to retract the entire lateral deltoid. We then insert a small or large pectoralis retractor medially (Fig. 1-5). We then mobilize the short flexors under the coracoid and place the pectoralis retractor deeper to retract these structures.

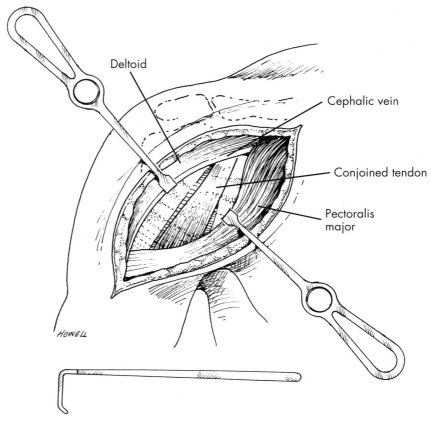

FIGURE 1-3

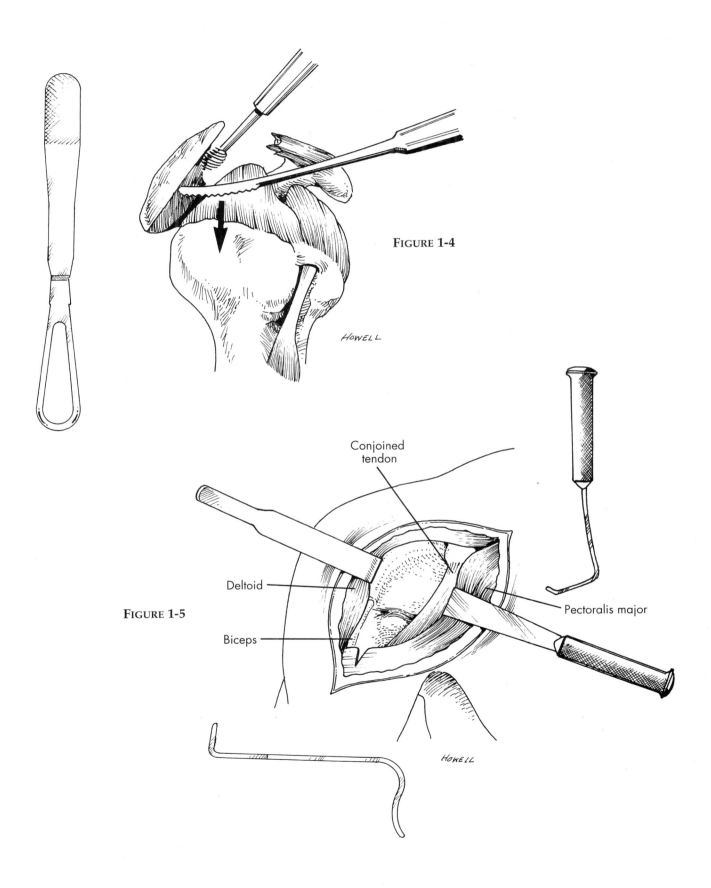

FIGURE 1-4

HOWELL

Conjoined
tendon

Deltoid

Biceps

Pectoralis major

FIGURE 1-5

HOWELL

In an anterior Bankart repair, after incising subscapularis and capsule, we insert a deep capsular retractor to pull the subscapularis and capsule medially and, with a humeral head retractor, retract or push the humeral head posteriorly. This procedure will allow visualization of the anterior glenoid rim (Fig. 1-6). We then retract the Bankart lesion medially with some form of anterior glenoid neck retractor, while leaving the humeral head retractor in place. This allows direct access for a surgical reconstruction of the Bankart lesion to the anterior rim. Fig. 1-7 shows the anterior soft tissue structures retracted medially with the anterior glenoral neck retractor. A larger humeral shaft retractor placed under the glenoid retracts the proximal humerus posteriorly, which is useful for hemiarthroplasty, total shoulder arthroplasty, or fracture reconstruction. This then allows access to the glenoid for the required surgery (Fig. 1-8). These retractors are applicable to most operative procedures, particularly in and around the glenohumeral joint.

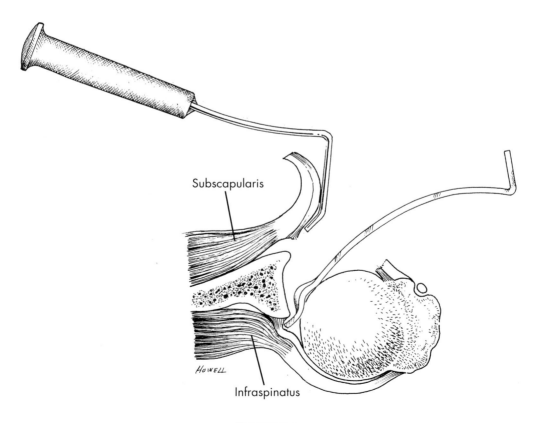

Subscapularis

Infraspinatus

HOWELL

FIGURE 1-6

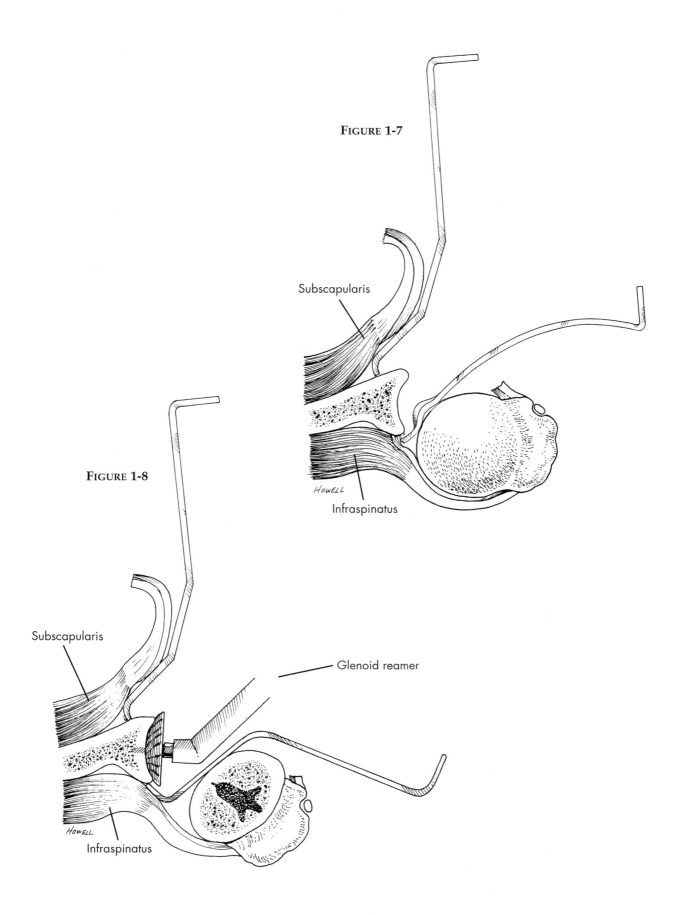

Figure 1-7

Subscapularis

Infraspinatus

Figure 1-8

Subscapularis

Glenoid reamer

Infraspinatus

Surgical Approaches

2

Introduction

There are many surgical approaches to the shoulder. With a better understanding of shoulder anatomy, current surgical approaches have evolved as primarily muscle splitting, thus avoiding the need to detach large muscles, such as the deltoid, from their origins. The surgical approaches in this chapter emphasize that principle and allow a rational understanding for performing the common shoulder reconstructive procedures.

In general, the skin incisions should parallel Langer's lines to allow better cosmesis with a fairly unremarkable scar. Even violating this principle does not lead to significant scarring unless a collagen abnormality is present. Incisions on the posterior aspect of the shoulder have a greater potential to result in some spreading of the scar. After the surgeon enters the deltoid through intervals, being careful not to violate tissue planes, the joint must be entered through the windows of deeper structures, such as the subscapularis and capsule anteriorly and the infraspinatus and capsule posteriorly. These muscle tendon units can be approached through muscle splitting avenues; however, incision of these tissues at right angles to their fibers is often technically easier and produces minimal disruption. The goal of current approaches is to minimize trauma, develop tissue planes, and allow an early aggressive rehabilitation program. The approaches that will be described are:

A. Anterior approaches
   1. Deltopectoral
   2. Extended deltopectoral
   3. Anterior superior
   4. Deltoid split
   5. Acromioclavicular

B. Posterior approach
   1. Deltoid split

C. Global approach

This chapter discusses the applications, indications, surgical techniques, and postoperative ramifications for each approach. We begin with a discussion of various positions used in these approaches.

Positioning
"BEACH CHAIR"

With most anterior approaches, the patient is placed in the "beach chair" position (Fig. 2-1). From the waist, the back, shoulders, and head are elevated in a straight line to approximate ly 30°. Nerves, along with pressure points, such as the ulnar nerves at the elbows, the peroneal nerves at the knees, and the posterior aspects of the heels, are protected. It is helpful to slightly flex the knees using a pillow and to strap the legs securely just above the knees so that the patient does not slide down on the table. The shoulder can be positioned near or even extending beyond the lateral edge of the table, depending on the procedure. Regardless of approach, a Steri-Drape around the neck to block saliva and hair from the wound lessens the chance of contamination. If desired, an inflatable cuff can be positioned under the ipsilateral scapula to bring the shoulder to an advantageous position and to allow adjustments during surgery. Appropriate draping of the entire upper extremity facilitates manipulation during surgery. An arm board may be used, depending on circumstances, assistants, procedure, and surgeon preference. Although not mandatory, a clear plastic drape over the wound holds the drapes in position and blocks out the axilla, a source of potential contamination. Some surgeons prefer to use a neurosurgical headrest for certain procedures, especially if a very superior approach is required.

SEMI-SITTING FOR OPEN AND ARTHROSCOPIC SURGERY

For open and arthroscopic approaches, a similar position can be used, with a greater degree of inclination of the upper torso to approximately 70° (Fig. 2-2). When performing arthroscopy, it is helpful to have a specialized back support to allow easy access to the posterior aspect of the shoulder. A patient under interscalene block will be able to control his or her own head, making this type of anesthesia practical for this position. Under general anesthesia, this position is less practical because the head must be secured with tape to the operating table, a somewhat compromised anesthetic situation. Performing arthroscopy in the sitting position allows conversion to an open procedure by simply lowering the table to the usual 30° upper torso inclination. This is usually done with the arm draped free so that no traction is used, perhaps a disadvantage in some arthroscopic situations.

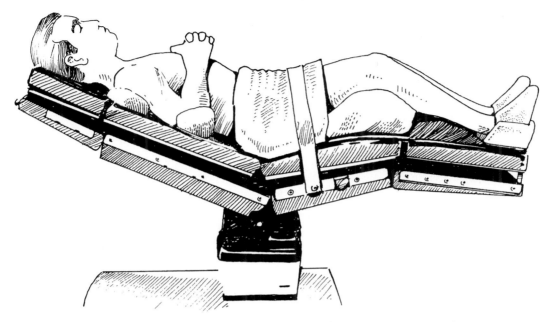

FIGURE 2-1

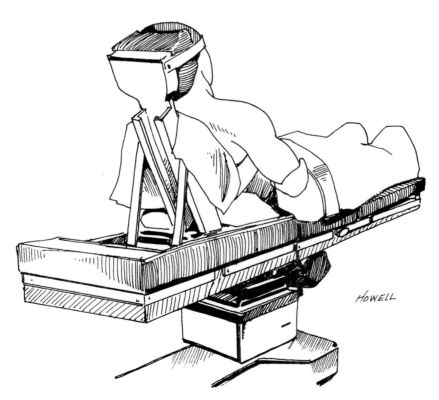

FIGURE 2-2

POSTERIOR OR PRONE

Posterior or prone positioning requires careful protection of nerves and pressure points (Fig. 2-3). Slight flexion of the knees and securing the body with a strap over the buttock or upper thighs is appropriate. The head must be carefully controlled by the anesthetist, ensuring protection of eyes and control of the endotracheal tube. The posterior aspect of the shoulder and the entire upper extremity can then be draped free to allow a more flexible approach and manipulation of the shoulder essential to most procedures.

LATERAL

The lateral position is used for arthroscopic surgery and for complex cases that may require both an anterior and a posterior approach, such as complex instability or fracture patterns (Fig. 2-4). Nerves, such as the peroneal, and pressure points, such as the greater trochanter, must be carefully protected. A Steri-Drape may be applied across the neck. Different positional holding devices, such as a kidney rest or a "bean bag," can be used to hold the patient in the lateral position. As in anterior and posterior approaches, the head and neck must be carefully supported. In the lateral position, the head must be kept in the sagittal plane to avoid excessive lateral flexion. An axillary roll may be placed in the down side axilla to protect neurological structures. With arthroscopy, a traction system should disperse stress throughout the upper arm with not too much weight, perhaps 8 to 10 pounds, and not too much abduction, perhaps 30° to 50° (Fig. 2-5).

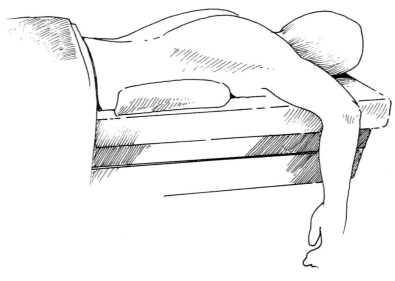

FIGURE 2-3

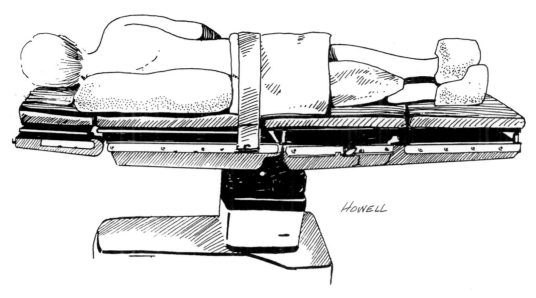

FIGURE 2-4

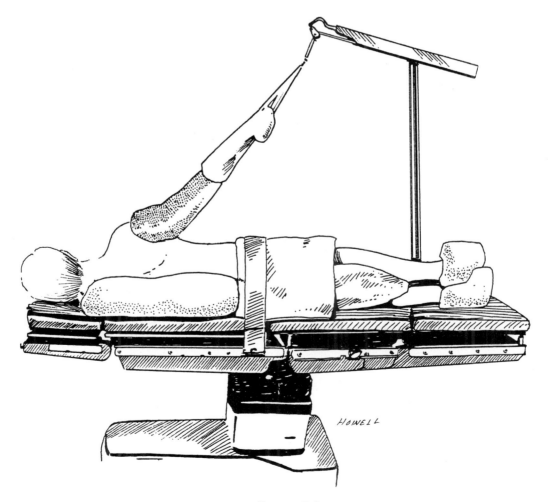

FIGURE 2-5

The direction of pull can aid in positioning the shoulder, which for arthroscopy would usually be approximately 30° inclined posteriorly to make the glenohumeral joint parallel with the floor (Fig. 2-6). If the shoulder is flexed 30° forward, the glenoid will not be parallel with the floor. It is important that the surgeon appreciate these features. For arthroscopic instability repairs, an additional traction system to distract the glenohumeral joint is helpful (Figs. 2-7 and 2-8).

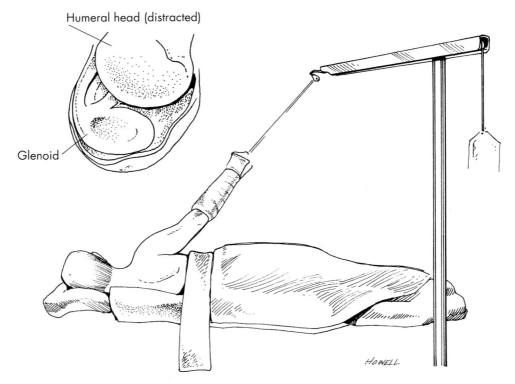

Humeral head (distracted)

Glenoid

HOWELL

FIGURE 2-6

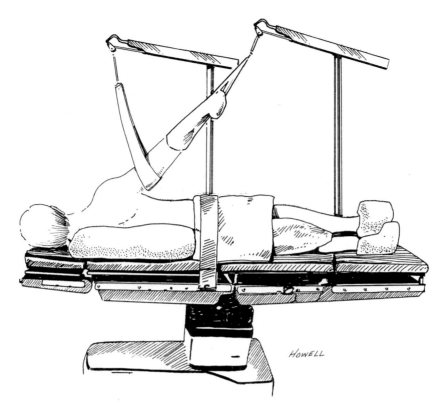

FIGURE 2-7

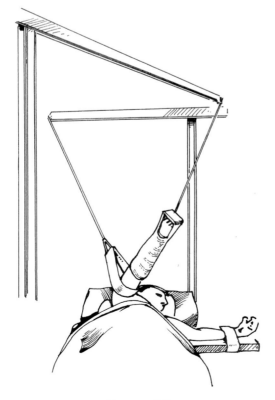

FIGURE 2-8

ANTERIOR APPROACHES

Deltopectoral

GENERAL CONSIDERATIONS

The most common situation in which a routine anterior deltopectoral approach is used is instability repairs, including Bankart and its modifications, Bristow, Putti-Platt, Magnuson-Stack, and Dutoit. This approach is also used for complex instabilities that use an inferior capsular shift and its modifications. This approach goes through the deltopectoral interval in which the cephalic vein lies. There is no violation of tissue planes.

SURGICAL TECHNIQUE

The patient is placed in the "beach chair" position with an inflatable cuff placed under the ipsilateral shoulder for slight elevation (see Fig. 2-1). If desired, this cuff can be positioned more toward the midline, causing the humeral head to be slightly anteriorly subluxated during part of the procedure. It can be deflated at the time of repair. The semi-sitting position is preferred by some surgeons (see Fig. 2-2). The approach is most often a routine anterior deltopectoral with an incision extending from just lateral to the tip of the coracoid, down to the axillary crease (Fig. 2-9). For cosmetic reasons, an axillary deltopectoral approach may be used. In this case, the incision may be started halfway between the coracoid and the axilla (Figs. 2-10 and 2-11).

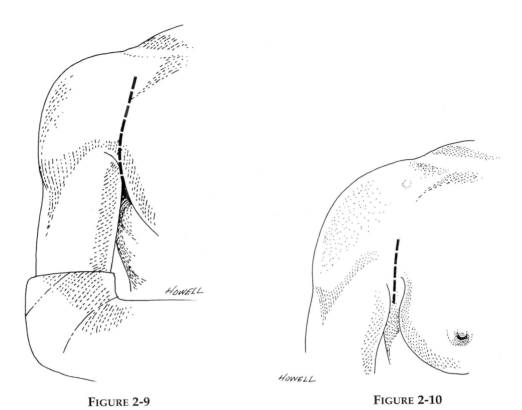

FIGURE 2-9   **FIGURE 2-10**

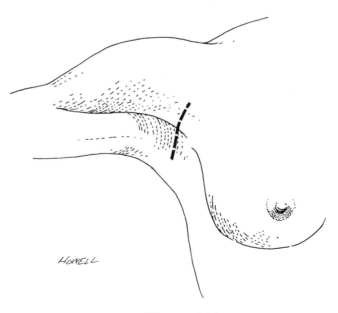

FIGURE 2-11

This axillary approach is similar to a routine anterior deltopectoral, but it requires more undermining to extend superiorly for the main part of the surgery. For cosmetic reasons, the incision can be positioned right in the axilla (Fig. 2-12). By laying the forearm across the chest and pulling upward on the skin at the level of the coracoid, one can get an appreciation of where the best cosmetic scar might be, which would be in one of the appropriate creases heading into the axilla (Fig. 2-13). After the arm is externally rotated to expose this area, the incision can be marked.

After the skin is incised and dissection taken down to the level of the deltoid and pectoralis muscles, gauze sponges can be used to spread subcutaneous tissue from its underlying muscle, and appropriate self-retaining retractors can be positioned for retraction, visualization, and initial hemostasis (Fig. 2-14). The cephalic vein is then identified, sometimes easily, sometimes not. The cephalic vein may be easier to identify where there is a slight separation of the deltoid and pectoralis as the vein approaches the acromioclavicular joint. Sometimes separating the deltoid at the interval of where the vein might be finds it in the depths rather than superficially.

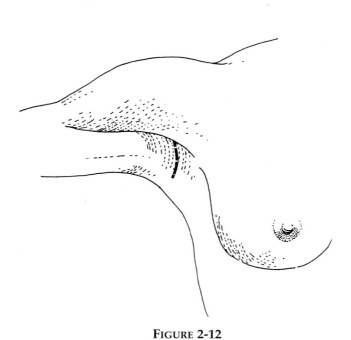

FIGURE 2-12

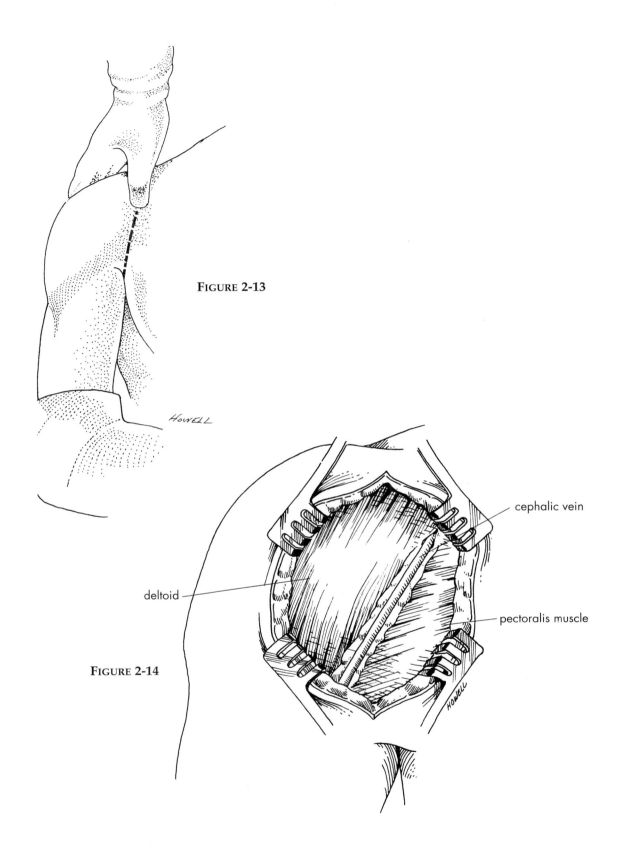

FIGURE 2-13

HOWELL

FIGURE 2-14

cephalic vein

deltoid

pectoralis muscle

HOWELL

Since most of the feeders come off on the deltoid side, the cephalic vein might be retracted laterally with the deltoid. With such a short approach, not too much retraction is used, so as not to endanger the cephalic vein, which can occur in an extended deltopectoral approach. By separating the deltoid and pectoralis muscles, the white clavipectoral fascia can be identified in the depths of the wound. The conjoined tendon is also visible (Fig. 2-15). With blunt finger dissection and traction, the subacromial space is freed up and a deltoid retractor is positioned to retract vein and deltoid muscle laterally and, if desired, superiorly. The pectoralis is retracted medially, with appropriate releases superiorly and inferiorly for exposure. The short flexors, consisting of brachioradialis and pectoralis minor originating from the coracoid, are identified. The clavipectoral fascia overlying these deep structures is incised, and a retractor is carefully placed to retract these short flexors medially, since the underlying musculocutaneous nerve is nearby (Fig. 2-16). The brachial plexus and axillary artery could also be jeopardized with overzealous retraction at this level.

Following these steps, appropriate identification of the biceps tendon, the subscapularis tendon with its insertion into the lesser tuberosity, and the supraspinatus tendon insertion above (Fig. 2-16) is possible. At this point, a decision is made as to how to enter the joint. Whether the subscapularis and capsule are separated and where capsular incisions are made will depend on the procedure and surgeon preference.

In principle, one might incise the subscapularis and capsule together, 1 cm away from the biceps and parallel with it (Fig. 2-17).

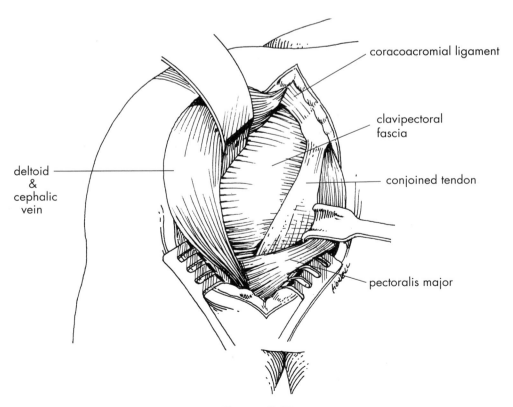

deltoid
&
cephalic
vein

coracoacromial ligament

clavipectoral
fascia

conjoined tendon

pectoralis major

FIGURE 2-15

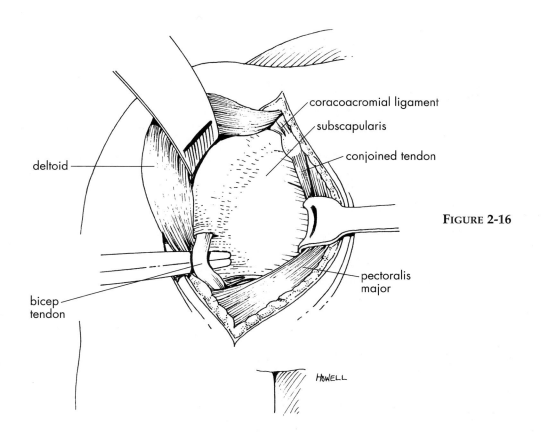

coracoacromial ligament

subscapularis

conjoined tendon

deltoid

bicep
tendon

pectoralis
major

FIGURE 2-16

HOWELL

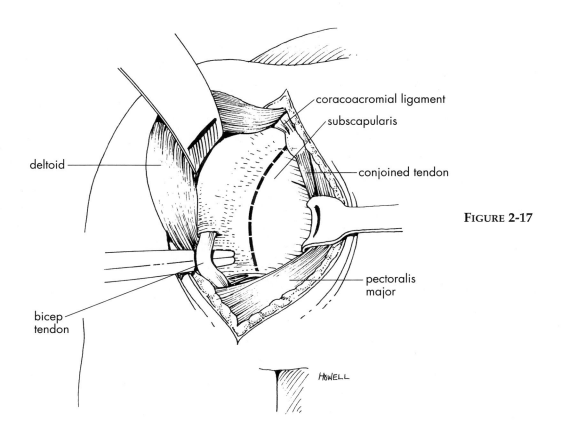

coracoacromial ligament

subscapularis

conjoined tendon

deltoid

bicep
tendon

pectoralis
major

FIGURE 2-17

HOWELL

Alternatively, one might wish to separate the subscapularis from the capsule, which can be achieved by various maneuvers. For example, beginning approximately 1 cm from the biceps, one might carefully incise the subscapularis at the musculotendinous junction, trying to leave the underlying capsule intact. Then with blunt dissection (Fig. 2-18) with a Cobb elevator, the subscapularis can be separated and retracted medially. One could also pass an instrument upward under the subscapularis from inferior to the interval above, only under muscle, hoping to leave capsule behind (Fig. 2-19). By then incising down on the subscapularis onto the underlying instrument, the subscapularis can be detached leaving the capsule intact. Even if one goes through both subscapularis and capsule together, they can still be separated with appropriate placement of stay sutures and careful dissection.

The subscapularis can also be split in the direction of its fibers at the junction of the middle and distal thirds, beginning more medially toward the glenoid where the underlying capsule is more easily identified. The capsule can also be incised in the same direction as the subscapularis split (Fig. 2-20). Muscle can then be separated from the capsule back toward its insertion and over toward and beyond the glenoid, which clearly exposes the underlying capsule.

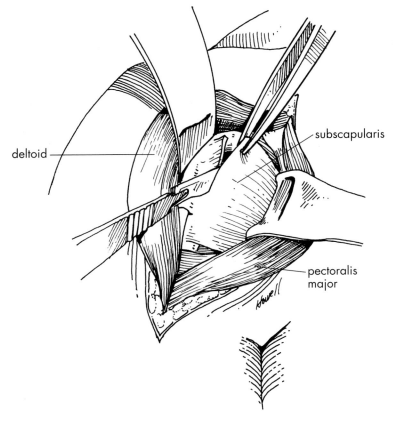

deltoid

subscapularis

pectoralis major

FIGURE 2-18

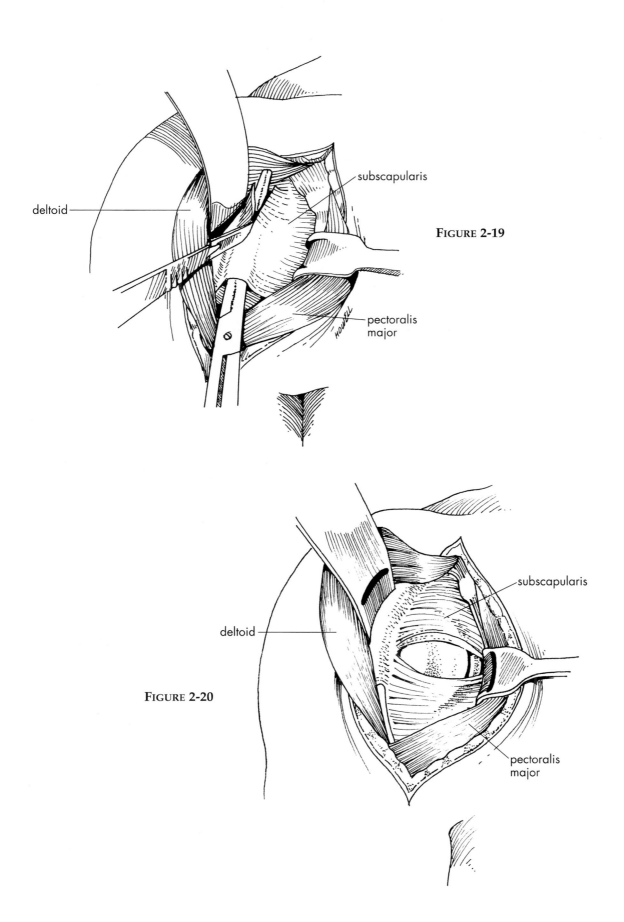

deltoid

subscapularis

pectoralis
major

FIGURE 2-19

deltoid

subscapularis

FIGURE 2-20

pectoralis
major

After the subscapularis and the capsule are separated, the next decision is how to incise the capsule to enter the joint (Figs. 2-20 and 2-21). The incision can be done laterally, centrally, or at the level of the glenoid in a vertical direction. It can also be done in a horizontal direction at different levels. The decision depends on the operative procedure to be used. For example, a modified Bankart repair can be done by incising the subscapularis and the capsule laterally, approximately 1 cm from the biceps, and repairing the capsule to the glenoid from within. Similarly, one can separate the subscapularis and the capsule, incise the capsule at the level of the glenoid, and perform a classical Bankart procedure as described by Carter Rowe. There are many modifications and each will be described with individual procedures. Reattachment of the capsule or reconstruction using this capsule and reapproximation of the subscapularis tendon depends on the procedure used. The subscapularis can often be reapproximated anatomically (Fig. 2-22).

Once the reconstructive procedure is completed, the deltopectoral interval simply falls back together requiring no suturing. Subcutaneous tissue and skin can be closed in the surgeon's preferred method. Because bleeding is minimal, using a drain is based on surgical preference but is seldom necessary with such procedures.

POSTOPERATIVE CARE

Postoperative care is simple because the violation of tissue planes has been minimal and there is no concern about protection, other than what might be related to the underlying reconstructive procedure. If the subscapularis has been violated, it may require some protection. From the perspective of this approach, usually immediate passive motion can begin, rapidly progressing to active motion and resisted exercises as pain permits.

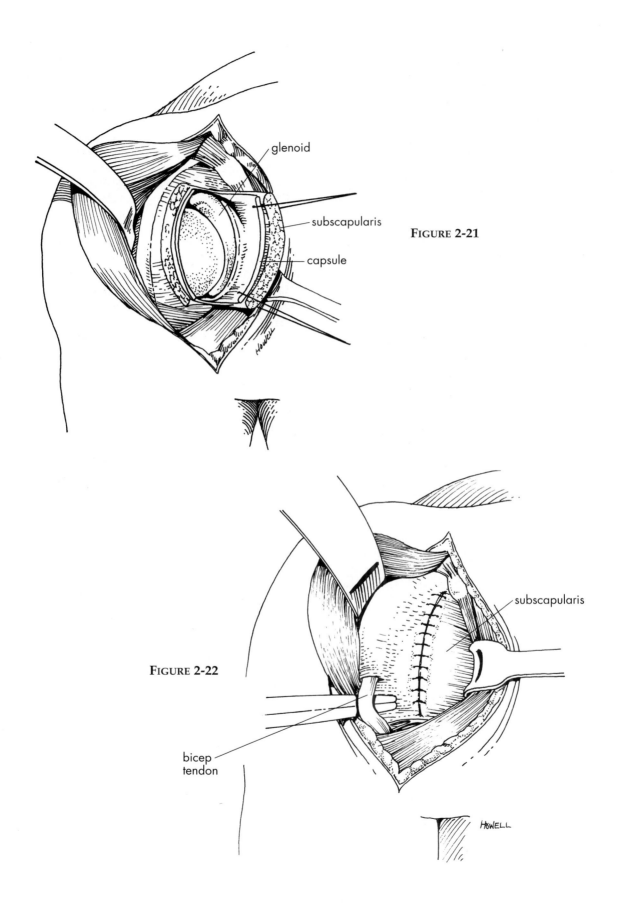

glenoid

subscapularis

capsule

FIGURE 2-21

FIGURE 2-22

subscapularis

bicep
tendon

Extended Deltopectoral Approach
GENERAL CONSIDERATIONS

The extended deltopectoral approach is a simple extension of the routine anterior deltopectoral approach, allowing a wider and longer exposure for an underlying reconstructive procedure, such as a total shoulder arthroplasty, hemiarthroplasty, fracture fixation, and other complex reconstructions. The principles of this approach are similar to the deltopectoral approach, only more extended, with release of more soft tissue for greater exposure.

SURGICAL TECHNIQUE

The patient is placed in the "beach chair" position (see Fig. 2-1) . An inflatable pillow can be placed under the ipsilateral shoulder. With a major reconstructive procedure, the glenohumeral joint should be at least at the level of the lateral edge of the table to allow appropriate posterior retraction without interference from the table top. The semi-sitting position is preferred by some surgeons (see Fig. 2-2).

The skin incision extends from the level of the anterior acromion down to the deltoid insertion. It can be gently curved, beginning at the medial acromion, heading toward the coracoid, and sloping down to the deltoid insertion (Fig. 2-23, *a*). The deltoid insertion is a considerable distance down on the lateral aspect of the upper arm. Alternatively, a straight incision may be used, extending from approximately the level of the acromioclavicular joint, passing lateral to the coracoid and down to the deltoid insertion (Fig. 2-23, *b*). Three self-retaining retractors are positioned, as in the deltopectoral approach, for exposure, visualization, and hemostasis (Fig. 2-24). The cephalic vein is identified and retracted with the pectoralis medially rather than laterally. This retraction creates some bleeding, requiring cautery. If the vein is retracted laterally, it frequently ruptures as a result of the excessive traction. If the cephalic vein is never identified, one must estimate where the interval is and go appropriately through that interval. After lateral retraction of the deltoid, a retractor is placed under the deltoid over the cuff in the subacromial space (Fig. 2-25). The pectoralis is retracted medially, the clavipectoral fascia is incised, and the short flexors off the coracoid are retracted, protecting the underlying vital structures. This allows identification of the biceps tendon, subscapularis tendon insertion, and supraspinatus tendon insertion. Exposure may be enhanced by releasing the overlying coracoacromial ligament. Release of the upper half of the pectoralis raphe is usually performed (Fig. 2-26).

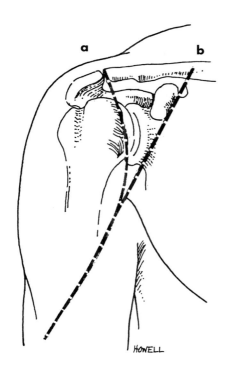

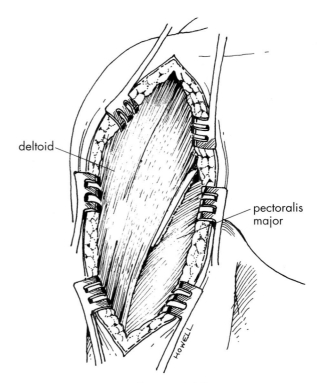

FIGURE 2-23

FIGURE 2-24

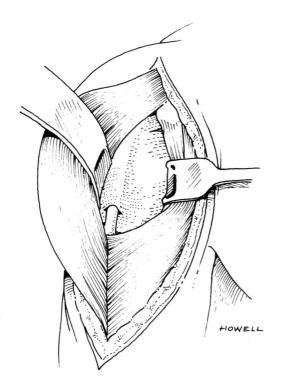

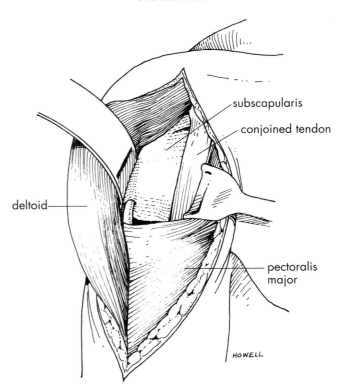

FIGURE 2-25

FIGURE 2-26

Part of the deltoid insertion can be released if there is excessive traction on the deltoid with retraction (Fig. 2-27). The arm can also be abducted to ease the insult to the deltoid musculature. In these procedures, it is probably not critical to repair the pectoralis raphe and deltoid insertions, but this can be easily achieved with simple sutures.

With a wide and long exposure, a decision can be made as to how to enter the glenohumeral joint or the fracture pattern can be identified. The subscapularis and capsule are frequently incised together at right angles to the biceps tendon, approximately 1 cm away from it, thus leaving a good cuff for reattachment (Figs. 2-28 and 2-29).

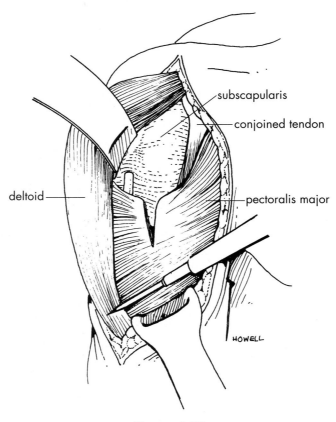

subscapularis

conjoined tendon

deltoid

pectoralis major

HOWELL

FIGURE 2-27

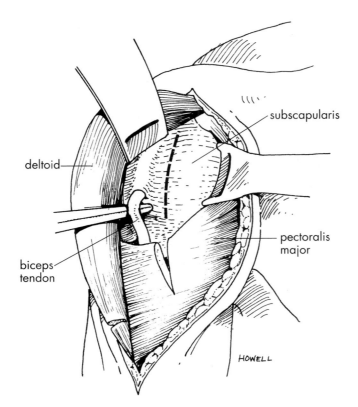

subscapularis

deltoid

biceps
tendon

pectoralis
major

HOWELL

FIGURE 2-28

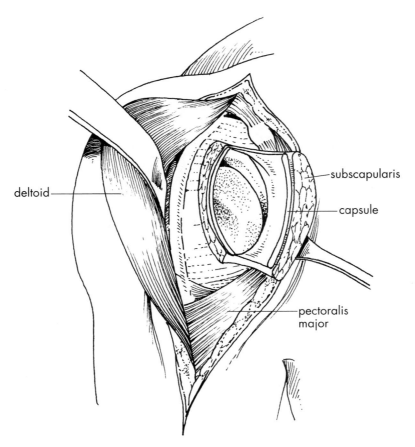

deltoid

subscapularis

capsule

pectoralis
major

FIGURE 2-29

In the presence of osteoarthritis with an internal rotation contracture, a Z-plasty lengthening of the subscapularis may be performed to improve postoperative external rotation (Fig. 2-30, *A*). Figure 2-30, *B* shows partial overlap, whereas Fig. 2-30, *C* shows end-to-end closure or greater lengthening. In fractures, the biceps acts as a landmark, allowing identification of the fracture pattern (Fig. 2-28).

POSTOPERATIVE CARE

Postoperative care is simple because the violation of tissue planes has been minimal and there is not much concern about protection, other than what might be related to the underlying reconstructive procedure. If the subscapularis is incised at right angles, it may require some protection in the postoperative period, especially protecting external rotation. Therefore, from the perspective of this approach, immediate passive motion can begin, rapidly progressing to active motion and resisted exercises as pain permits.

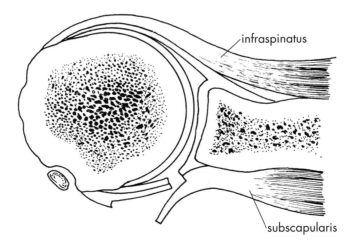

FIGURE 2-30 *A*

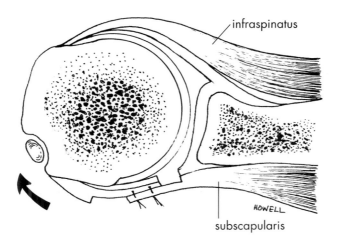

infraspinatus

subscapularis

FIGURE 2-30 *B*

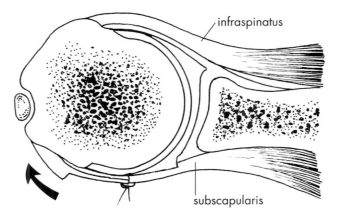

infraspinatus

subscapularis

FIGURE 2-30 *C*

Anterior Superior

GENERAL CONSIDERATIONS

The classic anterior superior approach was described by Neer in 1972 for anterior acromioplasty. The most common indication is to perform an open anterior acromioplasty with or without a rotator cuff repair. This approach can also be used for excision of calcium deposits or tissue excision of bursa and scar tissue. With this approach, the deltoid can be incised off the anterior acromion (deltoid off), or it can be split in the direction of its fibers (deltoid on), allowing side-to-side repair and perhaps more aggressive rehabilitation.

SURGICAL TECHNIQUE

The patient is placed in the "beach chair" position with an inflatable cuff placed under the ipsilateral shoulder (see Fig. 2-1). It is important to have the superior aspect of the shoulder well exposed near the lateral edge of the table and the head well out of the way. The semi-sitting position is preferred by some surgeons (see Fig. 2-2). The drapes must be positioned well up onto the base of the neck, allowing one to approach the shoulder from above.

It is appropriate to mark out the anterior and lateral acromion, the acromioclavicular joint, the clavicle, and the coracoid process to aid in positioning the skin incision. The skin incision is straight, but can be at different angles (Fig. 2-31). The importance of the incision is to provide access to the anterior acromion and the underlying deltoid attachment. This access can be achieved with an incision bisecting the acromion midway between the acromioclavicular joint and the lateral acromial border, extending over a distance of approximately 3 to 4 cm, one third above and two thirds below the anterior edge of the acromion (Fig. 2-31, *b*). Some prefer other modifications (Fig. 2-31, *a*).

Following the skin incision, the subcutaneous tissue and skin are appropriately retracted with self-retaining retractors for visualization and hemostasis. The white fibers over the anterior acromion and red fibers of the deltoid are identified. The anterior border of the acromion is visualized, palpated, and approached in a deltoid on or deltoid off manner.

The deltoid can be incised off the anterior acromion at right angles to its fibers, extending from the acromioclavicular joint to the lateral border of the acromion, a distance of approximately 2.5 cm (Fig. 2-32). It is helpful to leave a cuff of soft tissue over the anterior acromion for subsequent reattachment of the deltoid.

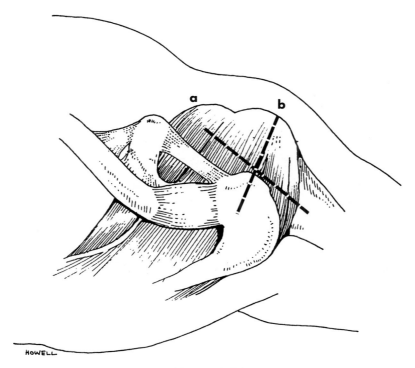

FIGURE 2-31

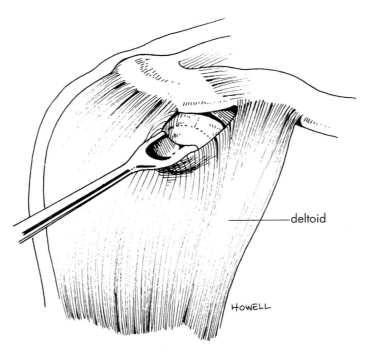

FIGURE 2-32

If a large rotator cuff tear is present and further exposure is required, the deltoid can be split distally, a distance of approximately 3 to 4 cm in the direction of its fibers, at the junction of the anterior and lateral aspects of the deltoid (Fig. 2-33). A stay suture can be placed distally to prevent propagation, which might interfere with axillary innervation of the deltoid.

The deltoid may also be managed by separating it in the direction of its fibers. This separation is achieved by extending the dissection up over the anterior acromion, spreading it subperiosteally off the roof of the acromion and distally into the deltoid (Fig. 2-34). Periosteal and fascial tissue should be obtainable on each side for subsequent reapproximation of the deltoid in a side-to-side fashion. The muscle can be separated at the lateral, mid portion, or medial aspect of the acromion. The deltoid fibers can be separated at the level of the acromioclavicular joint, extended distally, and by undermining the tissue, elevated in a sleeve-like fashion to allow fairly large reconstructive procedures, if necessary. This approach has been described by the Neviasers.

There are other methods of dealing with the deltoid. For example, its fibers can be incised at the anterolateral corner and over the top of the acromion in a transverse fashion, leaving a cuff of tissue anteriorly and posteriorly for subsequent reattachment.

Closure of the deltoid following these exposures depends on how it was initially managed. If incised off the anterior acromion, it can be either reapproximated to soft tissue, if there is a cuff remaining, or to drill holes in the acromion for secure fixation (see Fig. 4-13). If it had been approached in a side-to-side fashion, a side-to-side repair would be performed (see Fig. 4-14). If this is difficult to achieve, additional drill holes through the acromion may be required. Postoperatively, subcutaneous tissue and skin are closed in the surgeon's preferred fashion.

POSTOPERATIVE CARE

Some people are concerned that if the deltoid is incised off the anterior acromion, postoperative protection is required. Because such a small amount of deltoid is incised, it seems unnecessary for postoperative protection; therefore, either approach in handling the deltoid allows immediate passive motion, progressing to active motion and resisted exercises at a fairly rapid rate as pain and motion permit.

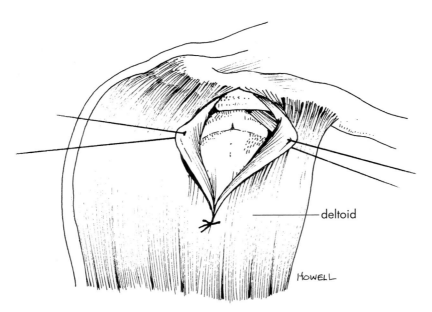

deltoid

FIGURE 2-33

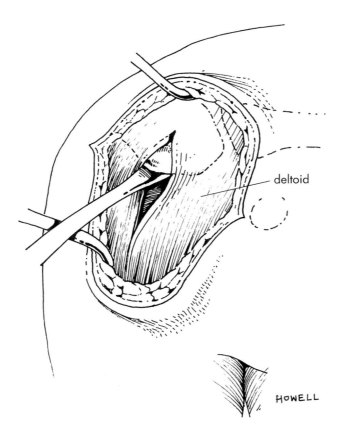

deltoid

FIGURE 2-34

Additional Deltoid Detachment

Sometimes in major reconstructive procedures, an additional part of the deltoid can be taken off the anterior and lateral acromion and the lateral aspect of the clavicle. In this case, it must be reattached to its origin. This reattachment can usually be achieved to a cuff of soft tissue; if not, then through drill holes in bone.

POSTOPERATIVE CARE

The postoperative care requires protection from active motion for approximately 6 weeks because of concern about deltoid detachment. During this time, passive or assisted motion can be performed. If a massive reconstruction is required, with a great deal of deltoid origin removed, an abduction pillow or brace may be required to protect the deltoid while it heals.

Deltoid Split

GENERAL CONSIDERATIONS

The main indications for using a deltoid split are a combined arthroscopic decompression and small, open repair of the rotator cuff or replacement of a greater tuberosity fracture fragment. Other indications include excision of calcium or a biopsy of small tumors in and around the rotator cuff or humeral head.

SURGICAL TECHNIQUE

The patient is placed in "beach chair" position with an inflatable pillow placed under the ipsilateral shoulder (see Fig. 2-1). The semi-sitting position is preferred by some surgeons (see Fig. 2-2). The deltoid split is centralized over the appropriate pathology and may vary as to whether it is anterior, lateral, or posterolateral. It is directly lateral in most circumstances. The skin incision can be a straight line in the direction of Langer's lines (Fig. 2-35, *A*) or at right angles to Langer's lines (Fig. 2-35, *B*); it need not be long. The subcutaneous tissue and skin are retracted, and the underlying deltoid is identified and split in the direction of its fibers to approach the underlying pathology. At the completion of the operation, the deltoid is simply allowed to reapproximate. The subcutaneous tissue and skin are closed in the surgeon's preferred fashion.

POSTOPERATIVE CARE

Because there is no violation of tissue planes, early passive range of motion can be increased to active and strengthening at a fairly rapid rate as pain and motion permit. Rate of progression may depend on the underlying reconstruction.

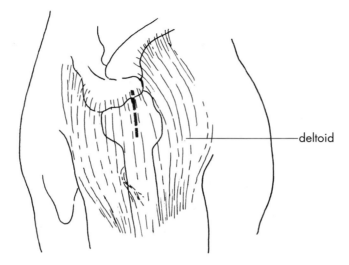

FIGURE 2-35 *A*

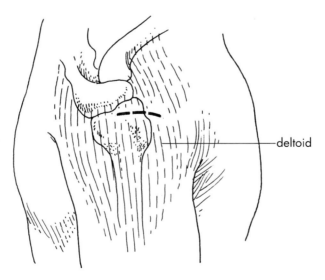

FIGURE 2-35 *B*

Acromioclavicular Approach

GENERAL CONSIDERATIONS

Three clinical scenarios necessitate an approach to the acromioclavicular joint or the outer clavicle: (1) excision of the outer clavicle, (2) fixation of the clavicle to the underlying coracoid, and (3) fixation of an outer clavicular fracture. Usually, a straight line incision can be used, but occasionally a curvilinear incision may be used if one is both approaching the acromioclavicular joint and attempting to fix the clavicle to the coracoid.

SURGICAL TECHNIQUE

The patient is placed in the "beach chair" position with an inflatable pillow placed under the ipsilateral shoulder (see Fig. 2-1). The shoulder must be lateral on the table, and draping must be appropriate for a very superior approach. The head must be well out of the surgical field; a cervical headrest would be helpful. The semi-sitting position for this approach is advantageous (see Fig. 2-2). Appropriate marking of clavicle, acromioclavicular joint, anterior acromion, and coracoid is performed. The skin incision for excision of the outer clavicle can be longitudinal in the direction of Langer's lines, oblique, or even transverse over the acromio-clavicular joint (Figs. 2-36 and 2-37). Self-retaining retractors allow exposure and hemostasis. The trapezial and deltoid aponeuroses are identified, and the acromioclavicular joint and overlying ligaments are incised, exposing the joint (Fig. 2-38). Subcutaneous tissue and skin are simply reapproximated at the end of the procedure based on the surgeon's preference.

Occasionally, an anterior acromioplasty is included with excision of the outer clavicle; thus the incision must allow access to both the anterior acromion and the outer clavicle.

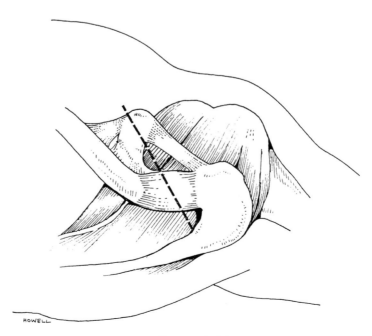

FIGURE 2-36

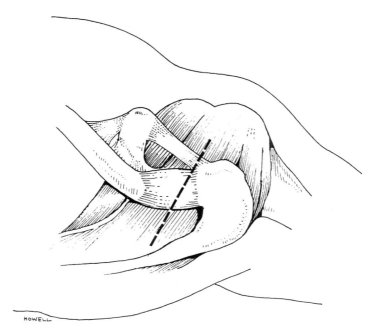

FIGURE 2-37

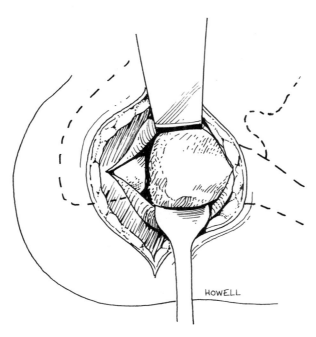

FIGURE 2-38

Several approaches can be used for fixation of the clavicle to the coracoid. For example, either a straight, longitudinal incision can be used or a curvilinear incision can be extended from posterior over the acromioclavicular joint and parallel with it, extending medially along the anterior superior border of the clavicle and extending in a curved fashion down to the coracoid (Fig. 2-39). In either event, the underlying deltoid muscle is identified and incised off the clavicle to identify the coracoid. The acromioclavicular joint can be identified through this approach. The deltoid may be reapproximated at the end of the procedure. Subcutaneous tissue and skin are closed in the usual manner.

POSTOPERATIVE CARE

Since tissue planes have been minimally violated, immediate passive motion can be implemented, progressing rapidly to an active and resisted program. When fixing the clavicle to the coracoid, or with pins fixing the acromion to the clavicle, we prefer to delay passive and/or active motion for 3 to 4 weeks until some healing occurs.

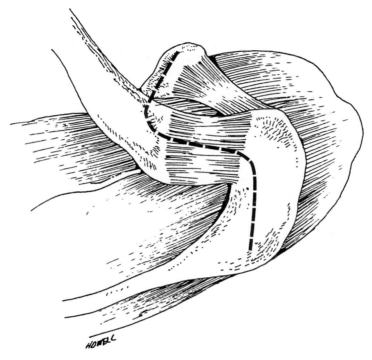

FIGURE 2-39

POSTERIOR APPROACHES

Deltoid Split

GENERAL CONSIDERATIONS

The posterior deltoid split is used primarily for stabilizing procedures for posterior shoulder instability or for an inferior capsular shift for multidirectional instability. Some fracture patterns can be reduced and fixed through this approach. Tumors are rarely approached in this fashion. The more extensive deltoid takedown from above or infraspinatus elevation from below are more applicable to certain fractures or tumors.

SURGICAL TECHNIQUE

For the deltoid split, the patient can be placed in either a prone (see Fig. 2-3) or, more preferably, a lateral position (see Fig. 2-4). The skin incision extends from the posterolateral aspect of the acromion toward the axilla, a distance of approximately 7 to 8 cm (Fig. 2-40). Subcutaneous tissue and skin are retracted with self-retaining retractors for hemostasis and exposure. The underlying deltoid muscle is identified (Fig. 2-41).

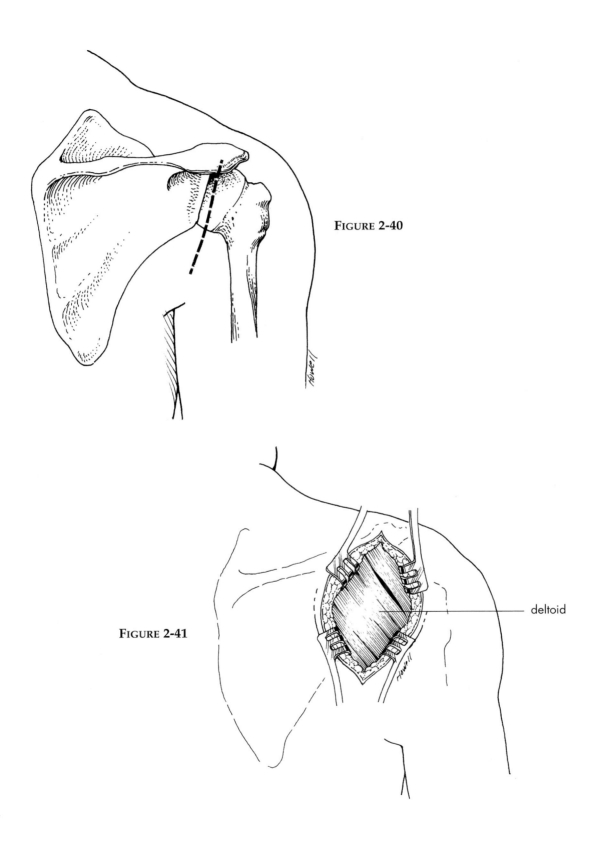

FIGURE 2-40

FIGURE 2-41

deltoid

The deltoid is split in its mid portion in the direction of its fibers and separated to identify the underlying infraspinatus and teres minor tendons (Fig. 2-42). The fibers of the underlying infraspinatus are identified by their different direction, almost at right angles to the deltoid fibers. In addition, an underlying deltoid fascia helps identify the next level. Appropriate retraction is placed and soft tissues released to allow adequate exposure to perform the required reconstruction.

The posterior aspect of the glenohumeral joint can be approached through a split between the infraspinatus and teres minor, or the infraspinatus tendon tissue can be incised at right angles to enter the joint (Fig. 2-42). The infraspinatus capsule can be entered horizontally. At the completion of the reconstruction, the deltoid simply falls back together requiring no sutures, and the subcutaneous tissue and skin are closed in the surgeon's preferred method.

POSTOPERATIVE CARE

Since no tissue planes have been violated with this approach, patients can begin immediate stretching and assisted exercises, progressing at a rapid rate to active and resisted exercises, taking into consideration the underlying reconstructive procedure.

More major posterior approaches will be described with management of scapular fractures.

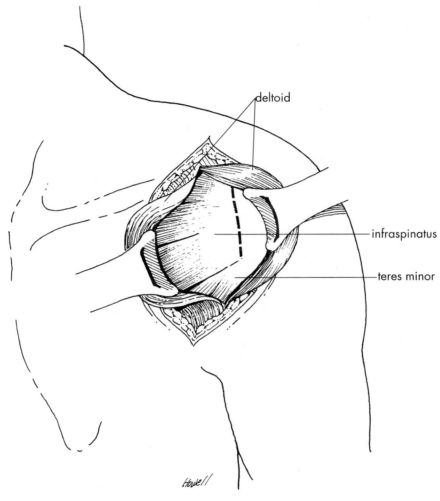

FIGURE 2-42

GLOBAL APPROACH

GENERAL CONSIDERATIONS

Occasionally, for resection of a tumor, amputation, or arthrodesis, a global approach to the shoulder is required (see Fig. 5-19). This approach violates tissue planes by requiring incision of the deltoid from its bony origin. It also violates underlying structures. The deltoid is incised from the anterior, lateral, and posterior acromion and reflected. This approach will be described with the appropriate procedures.

SURGICAL TECHNIQUE

The positioning for such massive exposure should usually be the lateral position to allow access to the anterior, superior, and posterior aspects of the shoulder.

The skin incision is variable, depending on the underlying pathology and approach. However, the incision often extends along the anterior humerus, over the superolateral aspect of the acromion, and along the posterior spine of the scapula. This incision is useful for arthrodesis. The underlying deltoid is identified and incised off the clavicle, acromion, and posterior spine of the scapula, allowing exposure to the underlying structures (see Fig. 5-19).

At the completion of the procedure, these muscles all require reattachment to their origin, which can prove difficult, compromising the postoperative rehabilitation by sometimes requiring abduction positioning of the extremity while these tissues heal. They can be repaired to a cuff of soft tissue and/or occasionally augmented with drill holes through their bony origin.

POSTOPERATIVE CARE

Because of the massive nature of the reconstruction and the violation of tissue planes, postoperative protection is required either in the form of positioning or by prohibiting active motion until healing has occurred. Passive motion may be allowed in the interim for 6 to 8 weeks, depending on the underlying reconstructive procedures.

Instability

3

Introduction

A reliable approach to instability problems is to first make an accurate diagnosis and then treat the appropriate pathology. The diagnosis of shoulder instability is usually straightforward and determined in the initial moments of the patient history. The more subtle forms of instability, such as in the throwing athlete or in the multidirectional patient, require a careful history and an extensive physical examination, using the apprehension sign, the sulcus sign, humeral head translation, and maneuvers such as the relocation test that aid in diagnosis. An appropriate classification of shoulder instability is based on direction (anterior, posterior, or multidirectional), frequency (acute versus chronic), etiology (traumatic versus atraumatic or overuse), volition (voluntary versus involuntary), and degree (subluxation versus dislocation).

The common causes of failure following surgery for shoulder instability are making the wrong diagnosis (that is, doing an anterior repair for a patient with multidirectional instability) and failing to correct the pathology (for example, failure to fix a large Bankart lesion). Other causes of surgery failure relate to hardware problems and making a reconstruction too tight. The latter event occurs with anterior instability, resulting in excessive compressive forces on the glenohumeral joint, or pushing the humeral head to a posteriorly subluxated position, both of which could result in osteoarthritis. A tight repair with limited motion is a significant functional disability, particularly in an athlete. The pathology seen with anterior instability varies, but can consist of a classical Bankart lesion with the labrum pulled off by the inferior glenohumeral ligament (Fig. 3-1, *A*), capsular stripping (Fig. 3-1, *B*), or capsular redundancy with an intact labrum (Fig. 3-1, *C*).

ANTERIOR APPROACHES
Bankart Repair (Classical)
GENERAL CONSIDERATIONS

The classical Bankart repair has been used for many years by Carter Rowe. It effectively compensates for the underlying pathology whether that is a Bankart lesion, a capsular redundancy without a Bankart lesion, or both. The subscapularis is separated from the underlying capsule, which is incised near and parallel with the glenoid rim and plicated in an east-west or medial-lateral fashion. If carefully performed, the repair allows maintenance of external rotation, even on the operating table.

Indications

The Bankart procedure is indicated for anterior instability of the shoulder with some type of Bankart lesion, most commonly with a traumatic etiology. A contraindication would be the presence of other instabilities, such as multidirectional instability. The pathology occurring in the different forms of instability varies. With traumatic anterior instability, there may be a classical Bankart lesion, capsular stripping, capsular redundancy, or some combination of these pathologies. Patients with multidirectional instability have a redundant inferior pouch. Patients with posterior instability have a lax posterior pouch and, rarely, a reverse Bankart lesion.

Expectations

The expectation following a Bankart repair is the elimination of the instability in a very high percentage of cases and return to full or near full external rotation. Some throwers may be able to return to their pre-injury level of throwing.

SURGICAL TECHNIQUE
Positioning

The patient is placed in the "beach chair" position with an inflatable pillow placed under the ipsilateral shoulder (see Fig. 2-1). The pillow may be placed toward the midline to allow the shoulder to lie in an anteriorly subluxated position during some of the procedure. The semi-sitting position is preferred by some surgeons (see Fig. 2-2).

Approach

The approach is an anterior deltopectoral or, if desired, an axillary approach for cosmetic reasons (see Figs. 2-9 to 2-11). The deltopectoral interval is identified, and the deltoid and cephalic vein are retracted laterally (see Fig. 1-15). The pectoralis and short flexors are retracted medially. The biceps tendon and its course are carefully determined (see Fig. 2-16). The subscapularis is approached and incised approximately 1.5 cm from a line parallel with the biceps tendon (see Fig. 2-17). The subscapularis is then separated from the underlying capsule (see Figs. 2-18 and 2-19) (see the anterior deltopectoral approach in Chapter 2 for methods of separation of subscapularis and capsule).

Procedure

The arm is positioned in slight external rotation, and the capsule is incised in a vertical fashion parallel with the glenoid rim approximately 2 to 3 mm from the rim (Fig. 3-2). The medial flap is elevated, and the pathology is identified.

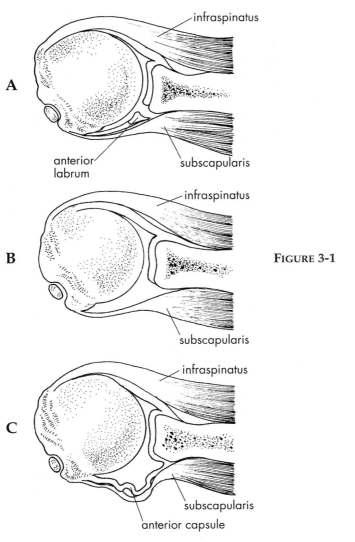

A

infraspinatus

anterior
labrum

subscapularis

B

infraspinatus

subscapularis

FIGURE 3-1

C

infraspinatus

subscapularis

anterior capsule

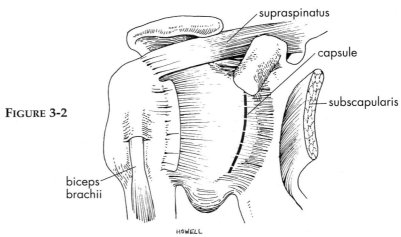

FIGURE 3-2

supraspinatus

capsule

subscapularis

biceps
brachii

HOWELL

The Bankart lesion and the capsule are then stripped from the glenoid neck, which is further decorticated. Three drill holes are made through the anterior rim of the glenoid for suture fixation. Alternatively, an anchoring system may be used through drill holes into the apex of the glenoid rim (Fig. 3-3). The lateral capsular flap is sutured down to the glenoid rim (Fig. 3-4). The medial flap is then sutured over the lateral flap using the same sutures in a pants-over-vest fashion (Fig. 3-5). Because the arm is in slight external rotation and the incision in the capsule is made near the glenoid, a significant amount of external rotation can be maintained. If the capsule is cut too far laterally and repaired as above, the shoulder could be made too tight, a significant pitfall.

Closure

The subscapularis is reapproximated from where it was originally detached (see Fig. 2-22). The deltopectoral interval is allowed to close (see Fig. 2-14), and the subcutaneous tissue and skin are closed as the surgeon prefers. A drain is not usually required, but this is left to the surgeon's discretion.

POSTOPERATIVE CARE (SEE CHAPTER 11)

A pressure dressing is applied, and the arm is positioned in a simple sling on the operating table. A strap around the abdomen, securing the sling and arm, will allow less movement during the early postoperative period and will lessen pain. Phase I can start on the first postoperative day, consisting of assisted elevation, internal rotation, and external rotation. External rotation should probably be limited to 30°, at the discretion of the surgeon. Pendulum exercises after a few days are an excellent warm-up.

Phase II begins at approximately 2 weeks, consisting of active elevation and internal and external rotation with terminal stretching. External rotation is limited to 45°. Elevation and internal rotation may progress to full rotation during this time. The sling is removed at approximately 3 weeks.

Phase III, which consists of concentric and eccentric rotational and anterior deltoid strengthening exercises, begins at 4 weeks, while continuing with the Phase II program. The sling can probably be removed between 2 and 4 weeks, at the discretion of the surgeon. In the athlete, scapular strengthening, such as shrugs and rows, can be added at this time.

By 3 months, full external rotation should be possible and the patient may resume normal activities, whether they include laboring work or sporting endeavors. Contact sports should be delayed until 4 months. Return to full training in an overhead athlete requires more time.

Bankart Repair (From Inside)
GENERAL CONSIDERATIONS

Performing a Bankart repair by entering the shoulder joint through the window of the subscapularis and capsule laterally avoids the difficulty of having to reach the glenoid rim from the outside. The approach has been described by Matsen in the *Journal of Bone and Joint Surgery,* and we have used it for 7 or 8 years. In general, the approach is to incise the subscapularis and capsule together in a vertical fashion, approximately 1 to 1.5 cm medial and parallel with the biceps tendon. By palpating and visualizing the joint at this point, the presence of a Bankart or a modification of the Bankart lesion can be determined. This procedure allows one to

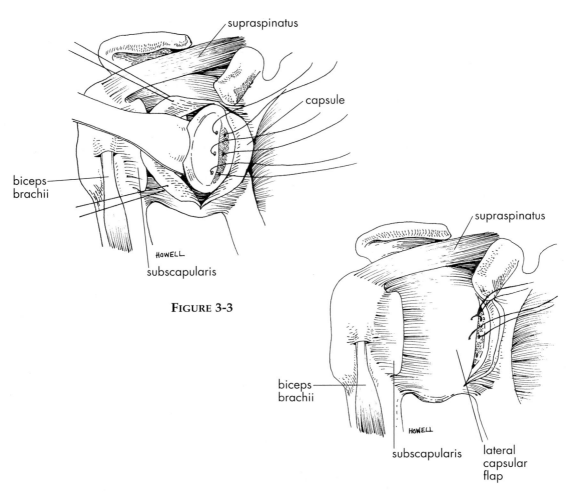

FIGURE 3-3

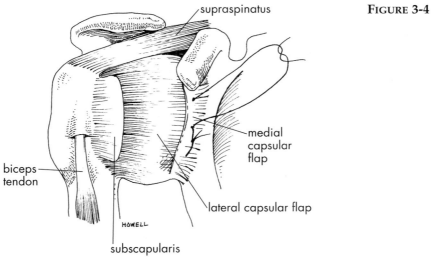

FIGURE 3-4

FIGURE 3-5

incise along the superior and inferior aspects of the subscapularis opening into the joint like a page in a book. This step allows easy access to the anterior glenoid, allowing preparation of the anterior rim to receive fixation for the Bankart lesion.

Once the Bankart lesion is fixed, the capsule and subscapularis can simply be reapproximated from where they were detached. This repair does not significantly violate tissue planes. It does, however, allow maintenance of external rotation. If there is no Bankart lesion, the subscapularis and the capsule can then be separated and an appropriate procedure can be performed, such as an anterior cruciate repair (described later in the text). Alternatively, a Bankart lesion could be created by detaching the labrum and then tightening it, taking some additional capsule to ensure stability. Or the capsule can be sutured to the labrum.

Indications

This repair has the same indications as the classical Bankart repair: anterior instability, which most commonly has a traumatic etiology with the presence of some type of Bankart lesion. It would be contraindicated in the presence of other instabilities, such as multidirectional instability.

Expectations

The expectations following this type of Bankart repair are the elimination of instability in a high percentage of cases and a return to full or near full external rotation.

SURGICAL TECHNIQUE
Positioning

The patient is placed in the "beach chair" position with a pillow placed under the ipsilateral shoulder (see Fig. 2-1). The pillow may be placed toward the midline to allow the shoulder to rest in an anteriorly subluxated position during some of the procedure. Some surgeons prefer the semi-sitting position (see Fig. 2-2).

Approach

The approach is an anterior deltopectoral (see Fig. 2-9), or if desired, an axillary approach for cosmetic reasons (see Figs. 2-10 and 2-11).

Procedure

The deltopectoral interval is identified, and the cephalic vein is retracted laterally with the deltoid (see Fig. 2-15). The pectoralis and short flexors are retracted medially. The biceps tendon and its course are carefully determined (see Fig. 2-16). The subscapularis and capsule are incised together, approximately 1 to 1.5 cm medial and parallel with the biceps tendon (see Fig. 2-17). The joint is opened vertically for a distance of approximately 2.5 cm at the junction of the lesser tuberosity and articular surface. The humeral head is pushed posteriorly to improve visualization, and with appropriate traction, palpation, or both, a determination can be made as to whether there is a Bankart or other lesion present.

If a Bankart lesion is present, an incision is made at the superior and inferior aspects of the subscapularis for a distance of approximately 4 to 5 mm, placing stay sutures at the superior and inferior corners to retract the flap medially. A humeral head retractor is then inserted into the joint to retract the humeral head out of the way (Fig. 3-6). A dinner fork–type retractor is placed under the Bankart lesion to expose the anterior glenoid rim (Fig. 3-7). If the Bankart lesion is incomplete, it can be enlarged with a Cobb elevator.

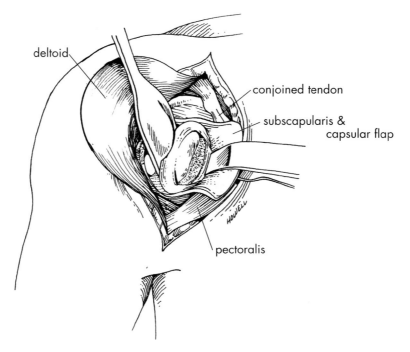

FIGURE 3-6

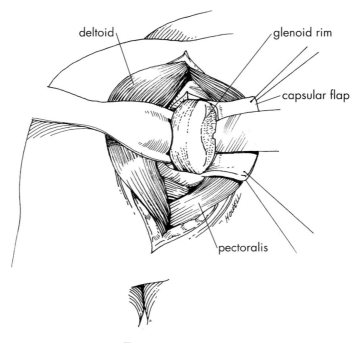

FIGURE 3-7

The anterior aspect of the glenoid is denuded down to cancellous bone to improve soft tissue healing to this area (Fig. 3-8). Three drill holes are made in the anterior rim of the glenoid for replacement of sutures (Fig. 3-9). A tenaculum, or towel clip (Fig. 3-10), can be used to ensure passage of sutures beneath the bony bridge from the glenoid surface to the anterior glenoid neck. Alternatively, an anchoring system may be used with drill holes into the apex of the glenoid (Fig. 3-11). Regardless of the means, sutures passed through the drill holes are then passed through the capsule at a position that will appropriately secure the capsule to the anterior glenoid face (Fig. 3-12). This is the critical part of the operation.

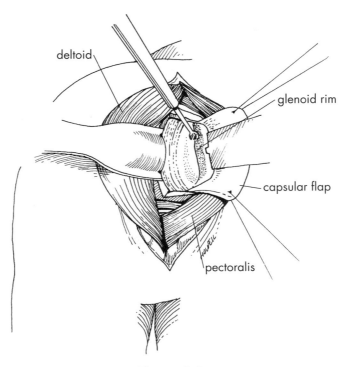

deltoid

glenoid rim

capsular flap

pectoralis

FIGURE 3-8

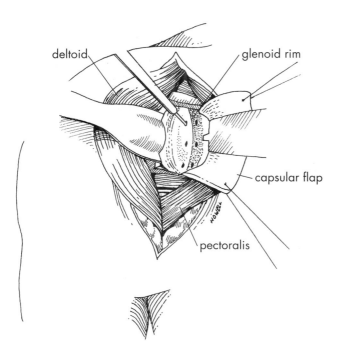

FIGURE 3-9

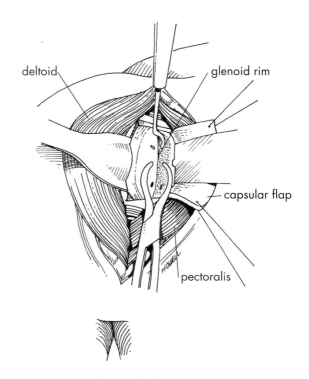

FIGURE 3-10

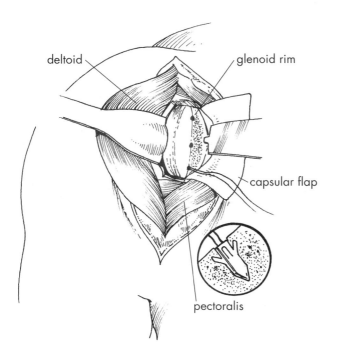

FIGURE 3-11

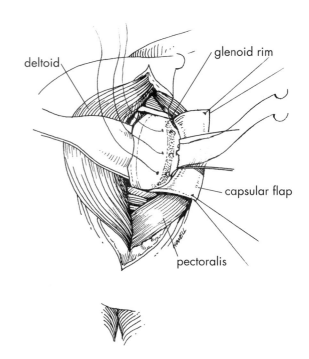

FIGURE 3-12

With traction on the stay sutures and an appropriate retractor positioned along the capsule, one can visualize where appropriate sutures should be placed in a simple fashion. Care must be taken when passing the suture through the capsule. If the suture is passed too deep into the subscapularis, "tightening and shortening of the subscapularis capsule may occur (Fig. 3-13). Only the capsule should be sutured, and only enough to eliminate the anterior pouch area, securing the Bankart lesion down to the glenoid rim (Fig. 3-14). Sutures are tied, and the subscapularis and the capsule are sutured into the position from where they were detached with no overlap (Fig. 3-15; see also Fig. 2-22). If added security is required, the capsule and the subscapularis can be overlapped laterally (Fig. 3-16). During suturing of the capsule medially, the position of the arm does not matter, but at the time of subscapularis and capsule closure laterally, it is important to ensure adequate external rotation before proceeding with the closure. If too much capsule is sutured or if some of the underlying subscapularis is captured, the repair can become too tight.

Closure

The subscapularis and the capsule are reapproximated from where they came (Fig. 3-15; see also Fig. 2-22). The deltopectoral interval is allowed to close (see Fig. 2-14), and the subcutaneous tissue and skin are closed as the surgeon prefers. The need for a drain is left to the surgeon's discretion.

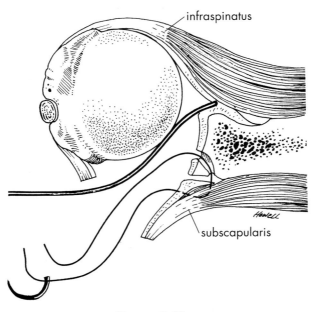

FIGURE 3-13

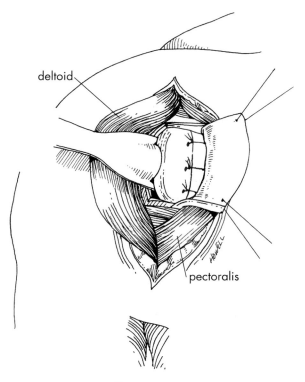

FIGURE 3-14

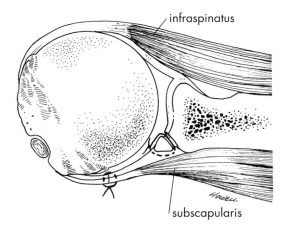

FIGURE 3-15

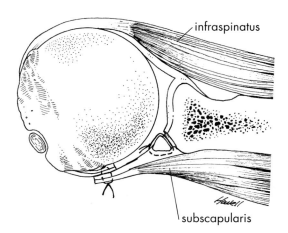

FIGURE 3-16

POSTOPERATIVE CARE (SEE CHAPTER 11)

A pressure dressing is applied, and the arm is positioned with a simple sling on the operating table. A strap around the abdomen securing the sling and arm will allow less movement during the early postoperative period and lessen the pain. Phase I can start on the first postoperative day and consists of assisted elevation and internal and external rotation. External rotation should be limited to approximately 30°, at the discretion of the surgeon. Pendulum exercises after a few days are an excellent warm-up.

Phase II, consisting of active elevation and internal and external rotation with terminal stretching, begins at approximately 2 weeks. At this point, external rotation should be limited to 45°. The sling is removed at approximately 3 weeks.

Phase III, which consists of concentric and eccentric rotation, along with anterior deltoid exercises, begins at 4 weeks, while continuing the Phase II program. External rotation is gradually returned to normal between 4 and 12 weeks.

By 3 months, full external rotation should be regained and the patient may resume his normal activities, whether in laboring work or sporting endeavors. Contact sports should be delayed until 4 months. Return to full throwing in an overhead athlete requires more time.

Bankart Repair (Subscapularis Split—Jobe)

GENERAL CONSIDERATIONS

The Bankart repair through a subscapularis split was developed by Dr. Frank Jobe for the throwing athlete. He believes that splitting the subscapularis rather than dividing it allows an easier and more effective rehabilitation program because the subscapularis is not violated. The Bankart repair is performed adjacent to the glenoid rim and requires medial exposure. This procedure is a modification of the classical Bankart approach performed through a subscapularis split, but more in a north-south or inferior-superior fashion. Postoperative immobilization in elevation and external rotation prevents scarring and diminishes eventual limitation of external rotation.

Indications

The indications are in a throwing or overhead athlete. Even in the absence of a Bankart lesion, such as with anterior capsular redundancy, this procedure is effective.

Expectations

The expectation for this procedure is elimination of the instability with return to maximal external rotation in a high percentage of cases and a reasonable chance of returning to aggressive overhead athletics, even throwing.

SURGICAL TECHNIQUE
Positioning

The position is "beach chair" with an inflatable cuff placed under the ipsilateral shoulder if desired (see Fig. 2-1). The cuff may be placed toward the midline to allow the shoulder to rest in an anteriorly subluxated position during some of the procedure. The semi-sitting position may be used (see Fig. 2-2)

Approach

The approach is anterior deltopectoral (see Fig. 2-9) or axillary (see Figs. 2-10 and 2-11). The deltopectoral interval is developed, and the cephalic vein and deltoid are retracted laterally (see Fig. 2-15), while the pectoralis and short flexors are retracted medially. The underlying subscapularis and biceps tendon are identified (see Fig. 2-16).

Procedure

With the arm in external rotation, the subscapularis is separated at the junction of its middle and lower thirds (Fig. 3-17) and spread to identify the underlying white capsular structure. With blunt spreading and separation of the capsule and the subscapularis, the capsule is widely exposed. The subscapularis fibers can be released laterally to the lesser tuberosity and medially over the face of the glenoid. With blunt dissection, this plane is easily developed and, with appropriate retraction, can allow a reasonable exposure. Specialized retractors are helpful in creating this north-south retraction of the subscapularis. A Homan-type retractor, placed both superiorly and inferiorly, and a modified Gelpi-type retractor will aid in retraction. The emphasis is on appropriate releases both laterally and medially to create a fairly long splitting of the subscapularis and to allow an extensile exposure of the underlying capsule (Fig. 3-18).

The capsule is then opened in line with the subscapularis split (Fig. 3-19). The pathology is identified, and the capsule may be incised vertically along the glenoid. The inferior flap is mobilized superiorly and the superior flap is mobilized inferiorly for an overlapping closure. We prefer not to incise the capsule parallel with the glenoid, but only parallel with the subscapularis split. Three drill holes are positioned in the anterior rim for placement of either sutures or an anchoring system, with the anchor being placed into the apex of the glenoid face and neck (Fig. 3-20). This better option of dividing the capsule only horizontally simply involves pulling the inferior flap superiorly and suturing it through two, if not three, drill holes in bone.

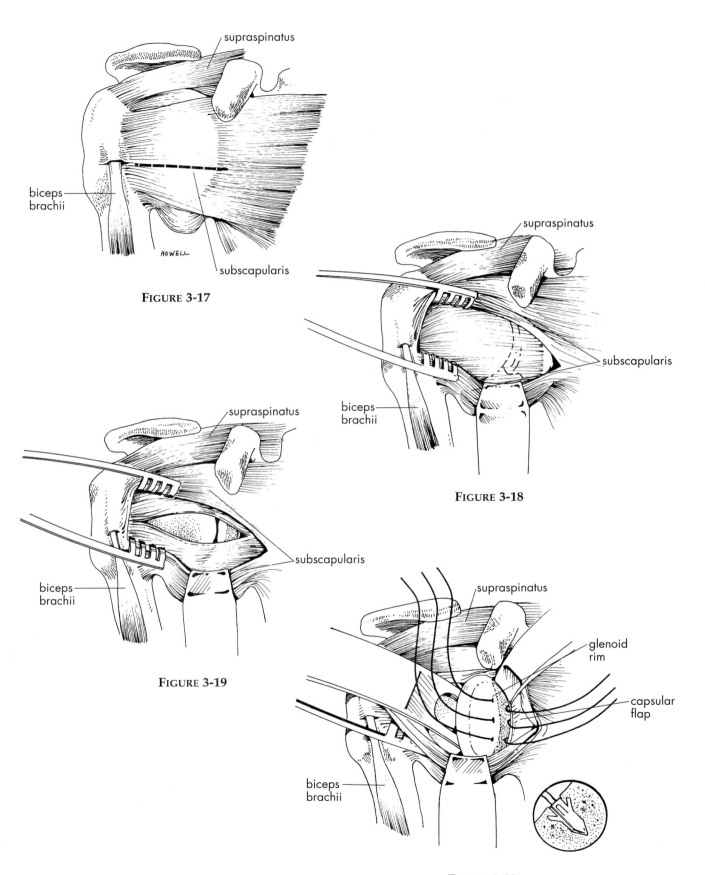

supraspinatus

biceps
brachii

subscapularis

HOWELL

FIGURE 3-17

supraspinatus

subscapularis

biceps
brachii

FIGURE 3-18

supraspinatus

biceps
brachii

subscapularis

FIGURE 3-19

supraspinatus

glenoid
rim

capsular
flap

biceps
brachii

FIGURE 3-20

Then, using the same sutures, the superior flap is tied down over the inferior flap in a pants-over-vest fashion (Figs. 3-21 and 3-22). This procedure creates a north-south rather than an east-west type of repair, as used in the classical Bankart procedure. This repair eliminates any Bankart lesion and any capsular redundancy. The repair is performed with the arm in external rotation to prevent compromise in the postoperative state. All of these sutures can be brought through both limbs of the capsule (Fig. 3-22). If less overlap is desired, only two sets of sutures are passed through both flaps (Fig. 3-23).

Closure

The subscapularis is then allowed to fall back together (Fig. 3-17) without the need for sutures. Similarly, the deltopectoral interval falls back together (see Fig. 2-14). Subcutaneous tissue and skin are closed as the surgeon prefers. The need for a drain is left to the surgeon's discretion.

POSTOPERATIVE CARE (SEE CHAPTER 11)

To prevent limitation of external rotation, the arm may be positioned for 3 weeks in an abduction splint, with the arm at approximately 45° external rotation. Exercises can be performed above the level of the splint, approaching full external rotation. The abduction rotation splint is optional, but an aggressive stretching program should still be emphasized.

The splint is removed at 3 weeks, and an active program is implemented, progressing to resisted exercises. In highly specialized athletes, return to sporting endeavors is delayed for 4 to 6 months. Throwing is not allowed for approximately 6 months and then only on a gradually increasing basis. In many cases, a full return to throwing may take up to 10 to 12 months.

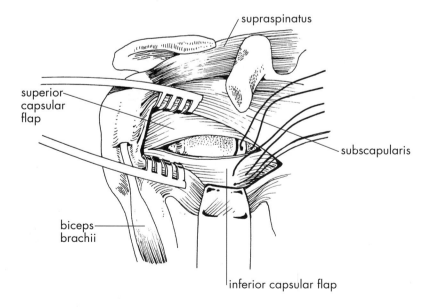

FIGURE 3-21

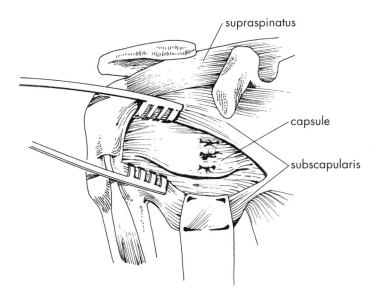

FIGURE 3-22

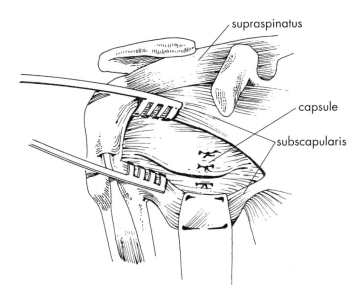

FIGURE 3-23

Anterior Cruciate Repair
GENERAL CONSIDERATIONS

This approach is modified from Neer and Foster's inferior capsular shift for multidirectional instability. It is an anterior capsular repair for anterior capsular redundancy and anterior instability. The repair is a north-south repair beginning at the level of the glenoid and extending to the lesser tuberosity.

Indications

The indications for this repair are best applied to the patient with anterior capsular redundancy without a Bankart lesion, that is, an intact labrum. This repair can be used with a Bankart lesion, but the Bankart lesion requires repair before performing the cruciate repair. This repair represents two procedures with some concern for potential restriction of motion caused by over-tightening. One must be careful to minimize this effect if using both procedures.

Expectations

The expectation following this procedure is similar to those following other stabilizing procedures for anterior instability: elimination of the instability with return of normal or near normal function and full external rotation.

SURGICAL TECHNIQUE
Positioning

The patient is placed in the "beach chair" (see Fig. 2-1) or semi-sitting position (see Fig. 2-2). An inflatable cuff may be placed under the ipsilateral shoulder. The pillow may be placed toward the midline to allow the shoulder to be partially subluxated during part of the procedure.

Approach

The normal approach is through the routine deltopectoral internal (see Fig. 2-9), although an axillary deltopectoral approach may be used for cosmetic reasons (see Figs. 2-10 and 2-11). The deltopectoral interval is developed (see Fig. 2-14), the cephalic vein and deltoid are retracted laterally, and the pectoralis and short flexors are retracted medially. The underlying biceps and subscapularis are identified (see Fig. 2-16). The subscapularis is separated from the underlying capsule (see Figs. 2-18 and 2-19) (see Surgical Approaches, Deltopectoral Approach for methods of separation).

Procedure

The subscapularis and the capsule are separated after an incision in the subscapularis is made approximately 1 to 1.5 cm medial to the biceps tendon. The capsule is also incised in a vertical fashion at this level for approximately 2.5 cm (see Fig. 2-17). There is often a superior interval or deficiency in the capsule that should be closed at this point (see Fig. 3-43). This same interval is closed with an inferior capsular shift. A lateral incision is made parallel with the biceps (Fig. 3-24). The capsule is then incised horizontally at a right angle to the initial cut (i.e., T'ed) down to the level of the glenoid (Fig. 3-25). The pathology is carefully identified. The best application of this procedure is, in the absence of a Bankart lesion, to eliminate the pathology of anterior capsular redundancy. Stay sutures are placed to retract flaps (Fig. 3-26).

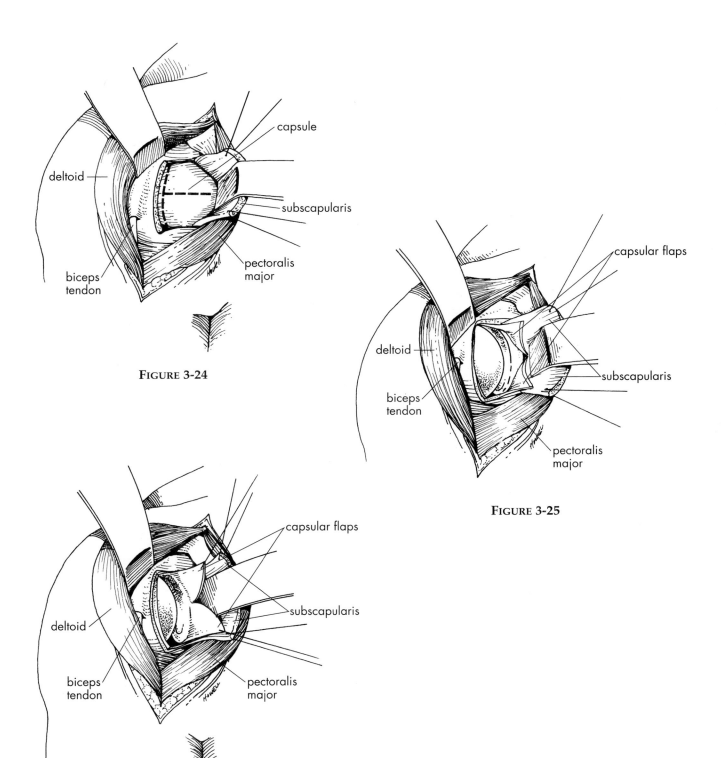

FIGURE 3-24

FIGURE 3-25

FIGURE 3-26

If no Bankart lesion is present, mattress sutures are placed, beginning at the level of the anterior glenoid rim in a north-south fashion, overlapping the capsule by no more than 4 or 5 mm (Fig. 3-27). Three or four sutures are then positioned, progressing laterally to the level of the vertical arm at the lesser tuberosity. As one proceeds more laterally, less overlap is possible, but there is less need for overlap at this level. The vertical arm of the capsule is then reapproximated from where it was detached (Fig. 3-28). The subscapularis is cosmetically reapproximated (see Fig. 2-22).

If a Bankart lesion is present, drill holes can be made in the glenoid rim (see Fig. 3-20), the Bankart lesion repaired, and the capsule sutured (see Fig. 3-23). Then, if desired, a north-south cruciate repair is used.

Closure

The deltopectoral interval is allowed to close (see Fig. 2-14), and the subcutaneous tissue and skin are closed as the surgeon prefers. The use of a drain is optional.

POSTOPERATIVE CARE (SEE CHAPTER 11)

A pressure dressing is applied, and the arm is positioned in a simple sling on the operating table. A strap around the abdomen, securing the sling and arm, will allow less movement during the early postoperative period and lessen the pain. Phase I can begin on the first postoperative day, consisting of assisted elevation and internal and external rotation. External rotation should probably be limited to 30° at the discretion of the surgeon. Pendulum exercises after a few days are an excellent warm-up.

Phase II is started at approximately 2 weeks, consisting of active elevation and internal and external rotation with terminal stretching. External rotation is limited to 45°. Elevation and internal rotation may progress to full rotation during this phase.

Phase III, which consists of concentric and eccentric rotation and anterior deltoid exercises, begins at 4 weeks, while continuing with the Phase II program. The sling can be removed between 2 and 4 weeks, at the discretion of the surgeon. In the athlete, scapular strengthening exercises, such as shrugs and rows, can be added at this time.

By 3 months, full external rotation should be obtained and the patient may resume normal activities. Contact sports are delayed until 3 months, and throwing is delayed an additional 3 months.

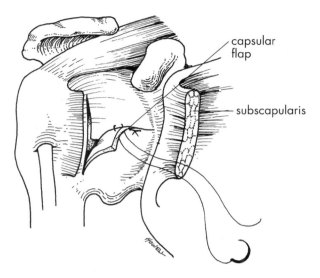

FIGURE 3-27

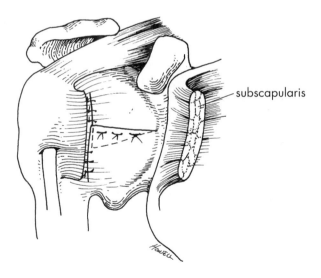

FIGURE 3-28

Lateral Capsular Subscapularis Advancement
(Modified Magnuson-Stack)

GENERAL CONSIDERATIONS

This operation does not address the pathology, but it can be used in the presence of anterior capsular redundancy, which is compensated for by lateralizing the capsule and subscapularis. Its application may be based on its technical ease.

Indications

It may be indicated in the presence of anterior capsular redundancy and the absence of a Bankart lesion.

Expectations

The expectations following this operation are the elimination of instability, functional return to activities, and in the long run, some limitation of external rotation. It is not designed for throwing athletes. Because it does not directly address pathology such as a Bankart lesion, there may be a slightly higher incidence of failure than in those that do correct the pathology.

SURGICAL TECHNIQUE

Positioning

The patient is placed in the "beach chair" position, with an inflatable cuff placed under the ipsilateral shoulder (see Fig. 2-1). The pillow may be placed toward the midline to allow the shoulder to rest in an anteriorly subluxated position during some of the procedure. The semi-sitting position may also be used (see Fig. 2-2).

Approach

The normal approach is an anterior deltopectoral (see Fig. 2-9), or an axillary approach may be used for cosmetic reasons (see Figs. 2-10 and 2-11). The deltopectoral interval is identified (see Fig. 2-14), and the deltoid and cephalic vein are retracted laterally (see Fig. 2-15). The pectoralis and short flexors are retracted medially. The biceps tendon and its course are carefully determined (see Fig. 2-16).

Procedure

Both the subscapularis and the capsule are incised at a right angle to their fibers, approximately 1 to 1.5 cm medial and parallel with the biceps tendon (Fig. 3-29). The incision extends from the plexus of veins below the subscapularis to just short of the interval above, a distance of approximately 2.5 cm. By pushing the humeral head posteriorly and retracting the flap, the underlying pathology can be identified. Incising the capsule in a transverse fashion at the superior and inferior margin of the subscapularis will allow easier identification of pathology and lateral advancement if indicated. If there is no Bankart lesion and only capsular redundancy, approximately 4 to 5 mm (Fig. 3-30) of capsule and subscapularis can be excised and the tissue reapproximated with simple sutures (Fig. 3-31). For a tighter repair, the subscapularis is overlapped (Fig. 3-32).

Closure

The deltopectoral interval is allowed to close (see Fig. 2-14), and the subcutaneous tissue and skin are closed as the surgeon prefers. The use of a drain is optional.

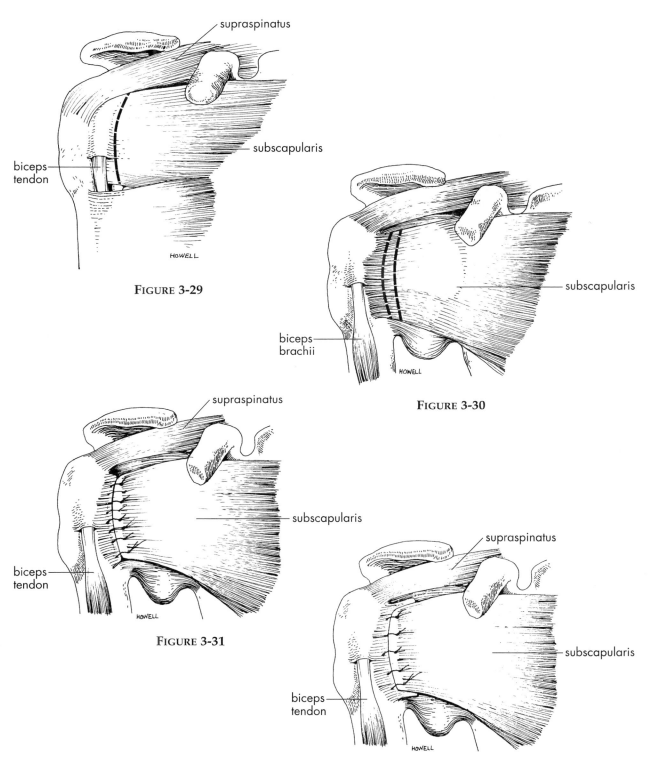

FIGURE 3-29

FIGURE 3-30

FIGURE 3-31

FIGURE 3-32

POSTOPERATIVE CARE (SEE CHAPTER 11)

Excising some of the subscapularis and the capsule causes concern about limitation of external rotation, which must be carefully addressed in the postoperative program. To ensure return of external rotation, more aggressive stretching can be used. The program can be the same as that employed under the inside out Bankart repair (described in that section).

Phase I can begin on the first postoperative day, consisting of assisted elevation and internal and external rotation. External rotation should probably be limited to 30°, at the discretion of the surgeon. Pendulum exercises after a few days are an excellent warm-up.

Phase II begins at approximately 2 weeks, consisting of active elevation and internal and external rotation with terminal stretching. External rotation is limited to 45°. Elevation and internal rotation may progress to full rotation during this phase.

Phase III, which consists of concentric and eccentric rotation and anterior deltoid exercises, begins at 4 weeks, while continuing with the Phase II program. The sling can be removed between 2 and 4 weeks, at the discretion of the surgeon. In the athlete, scapular strengthening exercises, such as shrugs and rows, can be added at this time.

By 3 months, full external rotation should be obtained and the patient may resume normal activities. Contact sports are delayed until 3 months, and throwing is delayed an additional 3 months.

Magnuson-Stack
GENERAL CONSIDERATIONS

The Magnuson-Stack, popular in the past, involves advancement of the sub-scapularis and the capsule from their insertion on the lesser tuberosity to the opposite side of the biceps, with stapling or suturing into the greater tuberosity. They are also advanced distally approximately half the width of the repair. This procedure obviously does not address the pathology, such as a Bankart lesion, but compensates by tensioning laterally. Some surgeons advance only the subscapularis, leaving the capsule intact.

Indications

The indication is for recurrent anterior instabilities, preferably, in the absence of a Bankart lesion.

Expectations

The expectations are for the elimination of instability in a high percentage of cases and return to reasonable functional activity, perhaps with some limitation of external rotation. Therefore, it is not applicable for overhead athletes.

SURGICAL TECHNIQUE
Position

The patient is placed in the "beach chair" position, with an inflatable pillow placed under the ipsilateral shoulder (see Fig. 2-1). The pillow may be placed toward the midline to allow the shoulder to rest in an anteriorly subluxated position during some of the procedure. The semi-sitting position may be used (see Fig. 2-2).

Approach

The normal approach is an anterior deltopectoral (see Fig. 2-9), or an axillary approach may be used for cosmetic reasons (see Figs. 2-10 and 2-11). The deltopectoral interval is identified (see Fig. 2-14), and the deltoid and cephalic vein are retracted laterally. The pectoralis and short flexors are retracted medially. The biceps tendon and its course are carefully determined (see Fig. 2-16).

Procedure

The subscapularis is incised directly adjacent to the biceps tendon and dissected medially off the lesser tuberosity over a distance of 2.5 cm (Fig. 3-29). The underlying capsule may be left intact (Fig. 3-33). Some surgeons also elevate the capsule. Superior and inferior transverse incisions, a distance of approximately 5 mm, are made in the subscapularis with stay sutures positioned at each corner. The greater tuberosity on the opposite side of the bicipital groove is denuded of soft tissue down to the bleeding bone. Alternatively, a trough may be created in an area approximately 1 cm distal to the tuberosity (Fig. 3-34). The subscapularis, with or without the capsule, is then advanced and either stapled to this position or sutured to a trough of bone, the latter being preferred (Fig. 3-35).

Closure

The superior interval is closed, the deltopectoral interval is allowed to close (see Fig. 2-14), and the subcutaneous tissue and skin are closed as the surgeon prefers. Use of a drain is optional.

POSTOPERATIVE CARE (SEE CHAPTER 11)

The postoperative program is similar to that used in the initial operative description of the inside out Bankart repair. The only exception is that because of the lateral advancement, one must be careful to aggressively stretch external rotation so as not to limit this motion.

Phase I can begin on the first postoperative day, consisting of assisted elevation and internal and external rotation. External rotation should probably be limited to 30° at the discretion of the surgeon. Pendulum exercises after a few days are an excellent warm-up.

Phase II begins at approximately 2 weeks, consisting of active elevation and internal and external rotation with terminal stretching. External rotation is limited to 45°. Elevation and internal rotation may progress to full rotation during this phase.

Phase III, which consists of concentric and eccentric rotation and anterior deltoid exercises, begins at 4 weeks, while continuing with the Phase II program. The sling can be removed between 2 and 4 weeks, at the discretion of the surgeon. In the athlete, scapular strengthening exercises, such as shrugs and rows, can be added at this time.

By 3 months, full external rotation should be present and the patient may resume normal activities. Contact sports are delayed until 3 months, and throwing is delayed an additional 3 months.

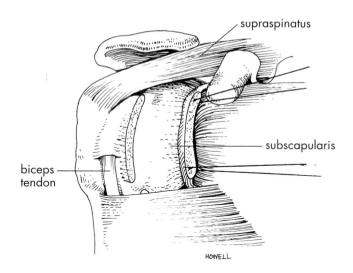

FIGURE 3-33

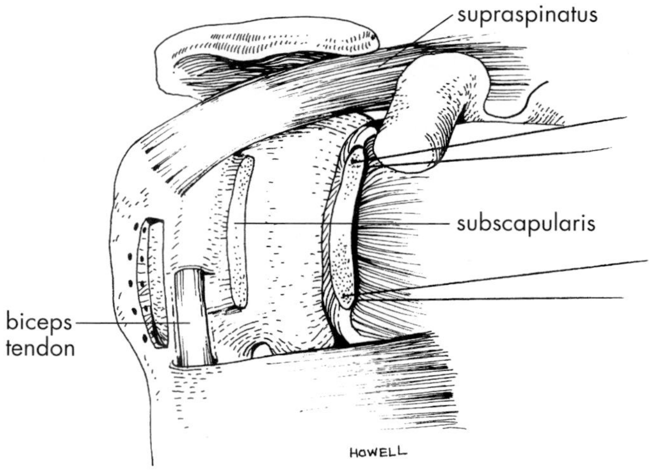

FIGURE 3-34

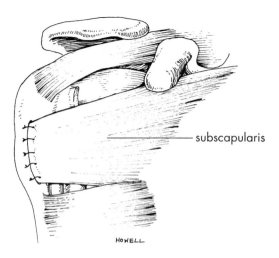

FIGURE 3-35

Putti-Platt Repair

GENERAL CONSIDERATIONS

The Putti-Platt is a standard repair for anterior instability but now is used less frequently, given our understanding of the pathology involved. The concern with the Putti-Platt repair is that it has a tendency or the potential to be made too tight, particularly in inexperienced hands. It can limit external rotation, resulting in limited motion and even osteoarthritis of the glenohumeral joint. If used, it must be done with precision and care so as not to make the shoulder tight, although this was the original intent: specifically, to limit external rotation by at least 25°.

Expectations

The expectation following Putti-Platt repair is that of elimination of instability in a high percentage of cases but with questionable return to a functional shoulder because of the limitation of external rotation that often results.

SURGICAL TECHNIQUE
Positioning

The patient is in the "beach chair" position, with an inflatable pillow placed under the ipsilateral shoulder (see Fig. 2-1). The pillow may be placed toward the midline to allow the shoulder to rest in an anteriorly subluxated position during some of the procedure. The semi-sitting position is preferred by some surgeons (see Fig. 2-2).

Approach

The normal approach is an anterior deltopectoral (see Fig. 2-9), or an axillary approach may be used for cosmetic reasons (see Figs. 2-10 and 2-11). The deltopectoral interval is identified (see Fig. 2-14), and the deltoid and cephalic vein are retracted laterally (see Fig. 2-15). The pectoralis and short flexors are retracted medially. The biceps tendon and its course are carefully determined (see Fig. 2-16).

Procedure

With the arm in approximately neutral rotation, the subscapularis and the capsule are incised in a vertical fashion, a variable distance from the glenoid rim (Fig. 3-36). The placement of this incision is critical to the success or failure of the operative procedure. If the incision is too close to the bicipital tendon, the repair will be too tight. It is appropriate to make the incision approximately 2 to 3 mm from the glenoid rim (Fig. 3-37). The detached lateral cuff of the subscapularis tendon and the capsule is then sutured to the anterior glenoid rim through drill holes (Fig. 3-38), and the overlapping medial flap of capsule and subscapularis is sutured in a pants-over-vest fashion (Fig. 3-39). One can appreciate the potential for this being a tight repair.

Closure

The deltopectoral interval is allowed to close (see Fig. 2-14), and the subcutaneous tissue and skin are closed as the surgeon prefers. The use of a drain is optional.

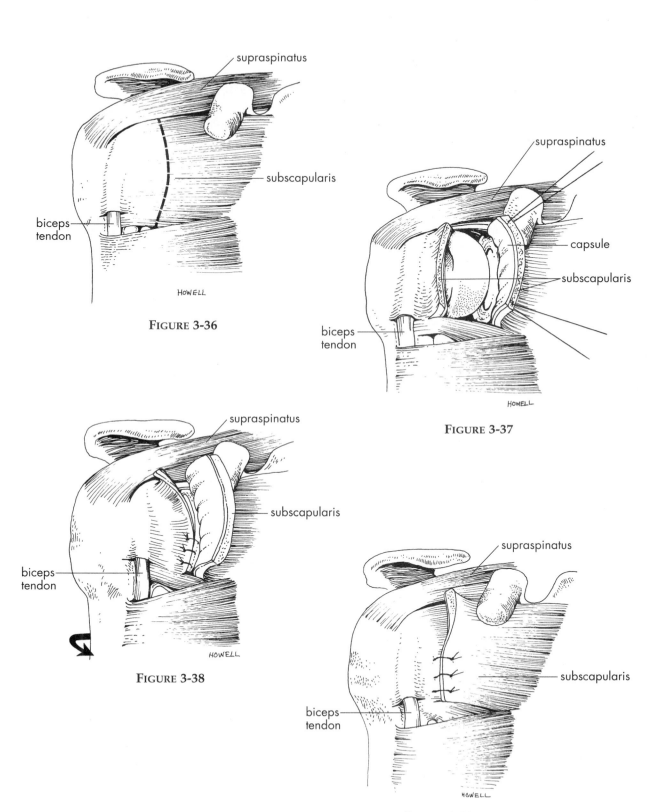

FIGURE 3-36

FIGURE 3-37

FIGURE 3-38

FIGURE 3-39

POSTOPERATIVE CARE (SEE CHAPTER 11)

Historically, these patients were immobilized for a period that increased the tendency toward subsequent limitation of external rotation. It would be appropriate to emphasize a very aggressive rehabilitation, particularly focusing on stretching external rotation as described under the inside out Bankart repair in the first part of this chapter.

Phase I can begin on the first postoperative day, consisting of assisted elevation and internal and external rotation. External rotation should probably be limited to 30°, at the discretion of the surgeon. Pendulum exercises after a few days are an excellent warm-up.

Phase II begins at approximately 2 weeks, consisting of active elevation and internal and external rotation with terminal stretching. External rotation is limited to 45°. Elevation and internal rotation may progress to full rotation during this phase.

Phase III, which consists of concentric and eccentric rotational and anterior deltoid exercises, begins at 4 weeks, while continuing with the Phase II program. The sling can probably be removed between 2 and 4 weeks, at the discretion of the surgeon. In the athlete, scapular strengthening exercises, such as shrugs and rows, can be added at this time.

By 3 months, full external rotation should be possible and the patient may resume normal activities. Contact sports are delayed until 3 months, and throwing is delayed an additional 3 months.

Bristow Procedure

GENERAL CONSIDERATIONS

The Bristow procedure is conceptually different from most anterior stabilizing procedures because it functions as a sling to prevent anterior translation of the humeral head as the arm is externally rotated and abducted. There is also obviously an element of scarring in the anterior capsule at the glenoid that results from this approach and further contributes to stability. The concerns with the Bristow procedure include the complications related to the osteotomy or to the use of hardware, along with the eventual tightness of the shoulder. There is also a higher failure rate with recurrence of instability and subluxation reported.

Indications

The indication for this procedure is recurrent anterior instability, regardless of underlying pathology.

Expectations

The surgical expectation is that of elimination of instability in a high percentage of cases, with some limitation of external rotation and some mild functional disability. There is a high failure rate for anterior subluxation. The Bristow has a higher rate of complications than the procedures that are designed to correct the pathology.

SURGICAL TECHNIQUE
Positioning

The patient is placed in the "beach chair" position, with an inflatable pillow placed under the ipsilateral shoulder (see Fig. 2-1). The pillow may be placed toward the midline to allow the shoulder to rest in an anteriorly subluxated position during some of the procedure. The semi-sitting position is preferred by some (see Fig. 2-2).

Approach

An anterior deltopectoral approach is used, (see Fig. 2-9), or an axillary modification may be used for cosmetic reasons (see Figs. 2-10 and 2-11). The subscapularis and biceps tendon are identified (see Fig. 2-16).

Procedure

The coracoid process is identified, and a small-diameter drill hole is placed in the tip of the coracoid process along its longitudinal axis. The coracoid is then osteotomized at a right angle to its axis with a segment approximately 5 to 7 mm long (Fig. 3-40). There are several ways to position the bone block, the attached coracobrachialis, and the short head of the biceps into the anterior glenoid area. It must be remembered that the bone block should be secured below the level of the equator of the glenoid. The subscapularis is split, and the bone block is positioned with a cancellous or cortical screw (Fig. 3-41). If a cortical screw is used, it should engage the posterior cortex of the glenoid. The inferior part of the subscapularis can be incised at the inferior glenoid, the bone block positioned, and the subscapularis reapproximated. Alternatively, the bone block can be passed beneath the subscapularis from inferior to superior and secured into the coracoid with a screw (Fig. 3-42). Once the bone block is secured, any soft tissue violation is repaired.

Closure

The deltopectoral interval is allowed to close. The subcutaneous tissue and skin are closed as the surgeon prefers. The use of a drain is optional.

POSTOPERATIVE CARE (SEE CHAPTER 11)

Exercises begin immediately and progress along the same program as described under the inside out Bankart repair, monitoring carefully the aspect of regaining external rotation.

Phase I can begin on the first postoperative day, consisting of assisted elevation and internal and external rotation. External rotation should probably be limited to 30°, at the discretion of the surgeon. Pendulum exercises after a few days are an excellent warm-up.

Phase II begins at approximately 2 weeks, consisting of active elevation and internal and external rotation with terminal stretching. External rotation is limited to 45°. Elevation and internal rotation may progress to full rotation during this phase.

Phase III, which consists of concentric and eccentric rotational and anterior deltoid exercises, begins at 4 weeks, while continuing with the Phase II program. The sling can be removed between 2 and 4 weeks, at the discretion of the surgeon. In the athlete, scapular strengthening exercises, such as shrugs and rows, can be added at this time.

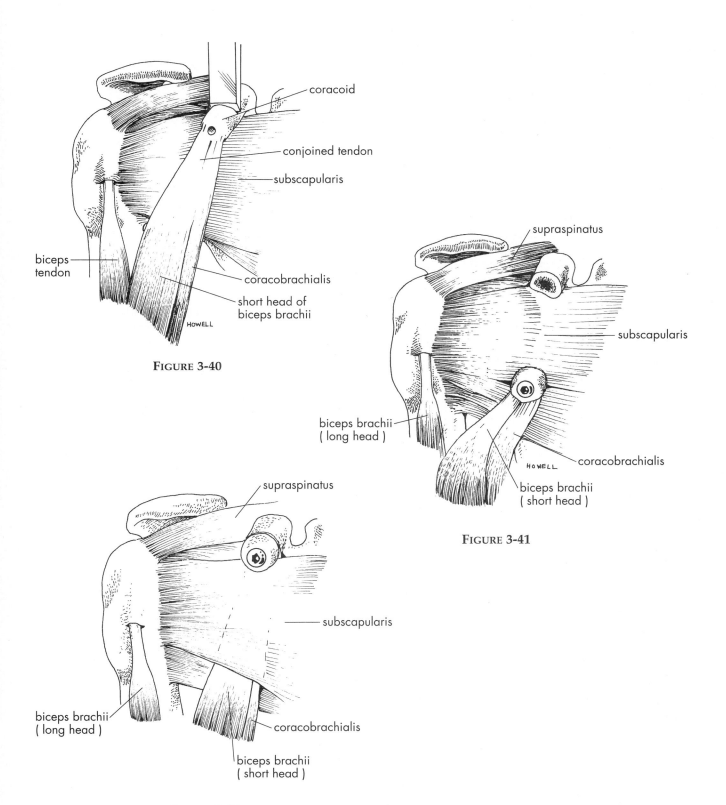

coracoid

conjoined tendon

subscapularis

biceps tendon

coracobrachialis

short head of biceps brachii

HOWELL

FIGURE 3-40

supraspinatus

subscapularis

biceps brachii (long head)

coracobrachialis

HOWELL

biceps brachii (short head)

FIGURE 3-41

supraspinatus

subscapularis

biceps brachii (long head)

coracobrachialis

biceps brachii (short head)

FIGURE 3-42

By 3 months, full external rotation should be possible and the patient may resume normal activities. Contact sports are delayed until 3 months, and throwing is delayed an additional 3 months.

Inferior Capsular Shift for Multidirectional Instability
GENERAL CONSIDERATIONS

The inferior capsular shift should be reserved for multidirectional instability and is most successful from the anterior approach. The diagnosis must be accurate. An inferior capsular shift is more challenging than other stabilizing procedures and was developed by Neer and Foster in 1980 to specifically address the defect of a redundant inferior pouch. These patients often have a collagen deficiency with loose joints, thus requiring careful attention to postoperative care with immobilization rather than stretching in the early stages. Many of these patients have had previous surgeries that have failed, adding to the complexity of the situation.

Indications

The indication for an inferior capsular shift is multidirectional instability of the shoulder. Many patients experience pain that often plays a major role in any operative decision. Many forms of multidirectional instability without pain can be easily tolerated with no long-term detrimental effects. In fact, the natural history of patients with multidirectional instability is that they will get better with time, if not subjected to surgery. Many surgeons use an inferior shift for routine anterior instability, which is acceptable, but it carries a different connotation than shifting for multidirectional instability.

Contraindications

The operation is of questionable value in other forms of instability, particularly anterior, because of a higher failure rate. It is also contraindicated as the only operation in a patient who has had multiple previous attempts at shifting procedures, or in a patient whose humeral head is inferiorly subluxated at rest. An inferior shift alone will be insufficient in these patients, and modifications are required.

Expectations

For the most part, expectations following an inferior capsular shift for multidirectional instability are to provide a stable shoulder that is functional for activities of daily living and light work. It is unusual for these patients to return to aggressive athletic endeavors. Unfortunately, there is a higher rate of failure with this procedure than in routine anterior procedures performed for traumatic instability. We have had a particularly high failure rate with multidirectional instability when approached posteriorly. Again, our present approach in these patients is to operate from the front.

SURGICAL TECHNIQUE
Positioning

For an anterior approach, the patient may be placed in the "beach chair" (see Fig. 2-1) or semi-sitting position (Fig. 2-2). An inflatable cuff may be placed under the ipsilateral shoulder. If there is any confusion regarding direction of instability, position the patient in the lateral position, allowing both anterior and posterior approaches if necessary (see Fig. 2-4).

Approach

The skin incision uses the deltopectoral interval (see Fig. 2-9) and can be modified with an axillary incision for cosmetic reasons (see Figs. 2-10 and 2-11). This is a difficult surgical exposure, and compromise by the use of an axillary incision should be minimized. The cephalic vein is identified (see Fig. 2-14) and retracted laterally along with the deltoid (see Fig. 2-15). Then the pectoralis and short flexors are retracted medially to identify the biceps and subscapularis tendons (see Fig. 2-16).

Procedure

The subscapularis is separated from the underlying capsule as described in Chapter 2 (surgical approaches—deltopectoral) (see Figs. 2-18 and 2-19). Beginning approximately 1 to 1.5 cm medial to the biceps tendon, the subscapularis is separated from the underlying capsule and retracted medially (see Fig. 2-17). The capsule is identified. Frequently, there is an interval superiorly between the middle and superior glenohumeral ligaments or between the superior glenohumeral ligament and the rotator cuff (Fig. 3-43). This interval requires closure to provide a base for the shift (Fig. 3-44). Reconstruction of the superior glenohumeral ligament, the coracohumeral ligament, or both, creating a superior sling, is an integral and important stabilizing part of an inferior capsular shift. The subsequent shift creates an inferior sling, eliminating the inferior pouch. At the same level that the subscapularis is incised, 1 to 1.5 cm medial and parallel with the biceps, the capsule is incised vertically for 2.5 cm (Fig. 3-45). This incision allows entry into the glenohumeral joint at the junction of the articular surface and the anatomic neck.

In the mid portion of the capsule, a horizontal incision is made down to the labrum on the glenoid rim (Fig. 3-46). Most patients who have multidirectional instability do not have a Bankart lesion. In the rare circumstances in which a Bankart lesion is present, it should be repaired in a conventional fashion before the shift is pursued. (See Bankart repairs for the various surgical options.) The inferior limb of the vertical incision is extended distally so that the capsule can be dissected from the humeral neck. With progressive external rotation, the capsule is dissected posteriorly. This dissection can be facilitated by the use of a Cobb elevator. Finger palpation allows one to determine whether the dissection has proceeded well around posteriorly to free up the entire inferior pouch. The principle behind working inside the joint is to provide protection for the axillary nerve by the intervening soft tissue. Knowledge of the anatomical course of the axillary nerve is imperative. If there is any element of excessive posterior play or any suggestion of posterior symptomatic instability in a patient with multidirectional instability, one must ensure complete posterior release from the humeral neck. With a finger in the inferior pouch, the inferior flap is pulled superiorly allowing for a determination of adequate tightness, based on the reduction of translation that has been achieved.

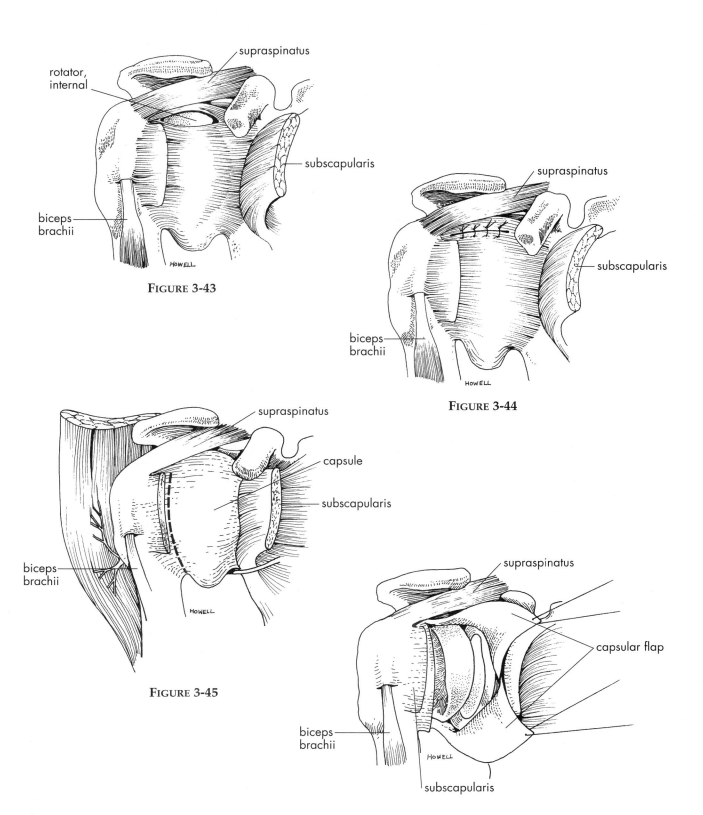

FIGURE 3-43

FIGURE 3-44

FIGURE 3-45

FIGURE 3-46

The subscapularis and the capsule are incised about 1 to 1.5 cm medial to the biceps tendon. Therefore, there is a margin of safety superiorly so that the cuff can be incised and a trough prepared in the nonarticular area of the lesser tuberosity. Superior and slightly lateral advancement of the inferior flap for 1.5 to 2 cm is performed, securing it to a trough just medial to the biceps tendon (Fig. 3-47). The first mattress suture securing the flap to the trough is critical, establishing the tension for the repair. This suture is positioned at the superior apex of the incision. Suturing is continued securing the flap to the lateral cuff of tissue, trying to mobilize it superiorly with each suture. This step creates both a superior transposition to eliminate the inferior pouch and some lateral transposition.

It is important to remember to reconstruct the coracohumeral ligament to provide a superior sling. The superior flap is then advanced distally and laterally and secured into soft tissue (Fig. 3-48). If there is further concern about anterior redundancy, sutures can be placed medially near the glenoid rim in a mattress fashion to eliminate any remaining anterior pouch redundancy (see Fig. 3-27). (See the anterior cruciate repair for anterior instability.) The subscapularis is then usually reattached to its original position. If there is a significant anterior component to the multidirectional instability, it may be laterally advanced (see Fig. 3-27).

Closure

The deltopectoral interval is allowed to close (see Fig. 2-14), and the subcutaneous tissue and skin are closed as the surgeon prefers. Use of a drain is optional.

POSTOPERATIVE CARE (SEE CHAPTER 11)

The postoperative care of a patient who has had an inferior shift for multidirectional instability differs from our usual instability rehabilitation. Unfortunately, in many of these collagen-deficient patients, the operation does not provide the desired ultimate security. The instability is complex. All of this suggests immobilization to add an element of scarring and security to the repair, which early mobilization may preclude. Therefore, the patient is immobilized in some form of shoulder spica cast or an appropriate orthosis for 8 weeks postoperatively. If there is concern that the patient may have more of an anterior instability than multidirectional, the immobilization period may be decreased. The position of immobilization depends on the predominant direction of instability. The key is to hold the humeral head against the undersurface of the acromion to allow the inferior pouch, as well as the superior reconstruction, to become secure. If the instability is predominantly inferior and anterior, the arm can be placed across the chest in internal rotation with the upper arm slightly anterior to the coronal plane. If it is predominantly inferior and posterior, the forearm should be in slight external rotation and the upper arm should be slightly posterior to the coronal plane of the body. If multidirectional instability is in all three directions, the upper arm should be in the coronal plane of the body and the forearm should be in neutral rotation pointing straight ahead. It is helpful to leave the axilla clear for hygienic purposes.

Following removal of the spica or orthosis, the patient is immobilized in a sling for 3 weeks.

Following immobilization in a sling for 3 weeks, an active rehabilitation program begins. Phase I is not performed because of the desire to eliminate stretching exercises from the program. The modification of the phasing is such that only active motion is begun, initially limited for the first month to 90° of elevation and 30° of external rotation and internal rotation to the belt line. It is unusual for stiffness to occur in these patients.

Inferior Capsular Shift Plus Coracohumeral Reconstruction Plus Nicola Tenodesis

GENERAL CONSIDERATIONS

Indications

For the multi-operated shoulder, particularly with failed attempts at inferior capsular shifts, and for the shoulder that sits inferiorly subluxated or dislocated, it may be inadequate to do only an inferior shift with the previously mentioned superior reconstruction. It will be necessary to emphasize the superior glenohumeral and coracohumeral ligament reconstruction and consider adding a Nicola-type tenodesis to stabilize the humeral head superiorly and anteriorly, particularly in the presence of an element of posterior instability.

Expectations

The expectations following this surgery are very limited in that the goal is to increase stabilization of the humeral head to lessen the symptoms of pain and disability. The failure rate following this procedure is high in the multi-operated shoulder because of the many failed operations and because the tissue is scarred and collagen deficient. The alternative to this procedure in the very painful shoulder may be arthrodesis.

SURGICAL TECHNIQUE
Positioning

The patient is placed in the "beach chair" position with an inflatable pillow placed under the ipsilateral shoulder (see Fig. 2-1). The semi-sitting position is preferred by some (see Fig. 2-2). The pillow may be placed toward the midline to allow the shoulder to rest in an anteriorly subluxated position during some of the procedure. The lateral position allows flexibility, should there be any need to approach anteriorly and posteriorly (see Fig. 2-4).

Approach

The skin incision uses the deltopectoral approach (see Fig. 2-9) or an axillary deltopectoral for cosmetic reasons (see Figs. 2-10 and 2-11). This is a difficult surgical exposure, and compromise with an axillary incision should be minimized. The cephalic interval is identified (see Fig. 2-14) and retracted laterally along with the deltoid (see Fig. 2-15). The pectoralis and short flexors are retracted medially, and the biceps and subscapularis tendons are identified (see Fig. 2-16).

Procedure

The capsule is split down to the glenoid. The subscapularis is incised 1.5 cm from the biceps, in line with the biceps, then resected off of the capsule. The biceps tendon is then identified in its groove and is incised at the distal extent of the groove (Fig. 3-49). A drill hole is made in the bicipital groove, exiting at the junction of the articular and nonarticular surface in the humeral head (Fig. 3-50). The inferior flap is advanced superiorly and sutured to soft tissue or a trough (see the section on multidirectional instability inferior capsular shift) (Fig. 3-51).

The detached tendon is passed from above through the humeral head and pulled securely anteriorly and stapled onto the bicipital groove, holding the head superiorly and anteriorly (Fig. 3-52). The superior flap is advanced and sutured inferiorly (see the section on inferior capsular shift) (Fig. 3-53).

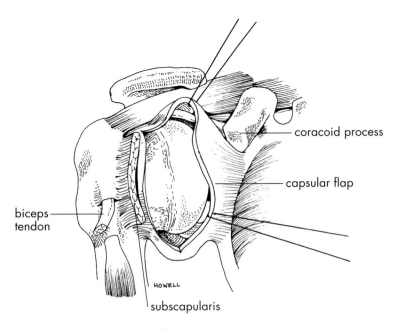

FIGURE 3-49

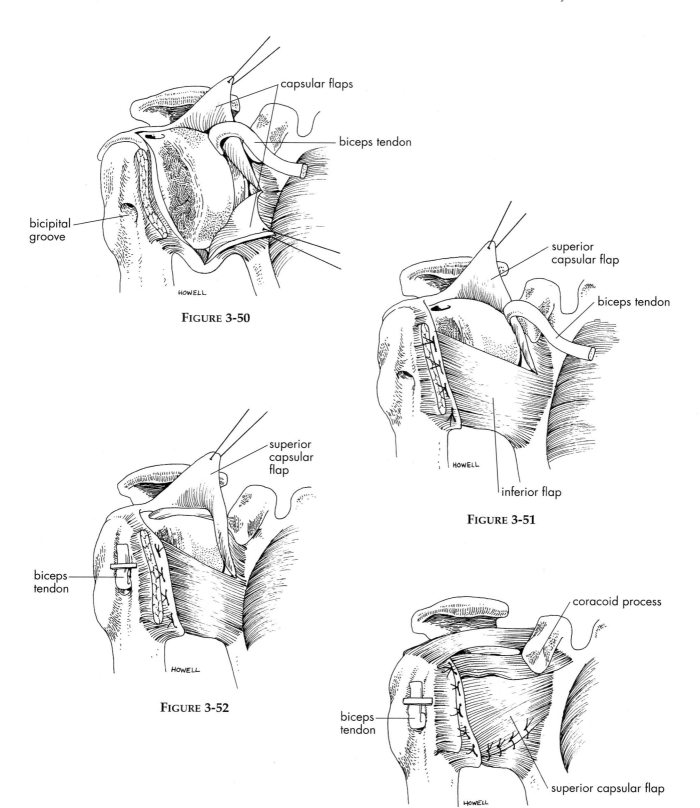

FIGURE 3-50

FIGURE 3-51

FIGURE 3-52

FIGURE 3-53

Large, strong sutures are passed through soft tissue at the base of the coracoid, down to the rotator interval, creating a coracohumeral-type restraint (Fig. 3-54). Mersilene, fascia, or palmaris longus tendon graft can be passed through the base of the coracoid and through the humeral head as a more dramatic stabilizing step. This pulls the humeral head anteriorly and, more importantly, superiorly. The inferior shift is performed before these two steps, which significantly diminishes translation of the humeral head, almost aiming toward a fibrous arthrodesis.

Closure

The subscapularis is reapproximated to where it was taken down (see Fig. 2-22). The deltopectoral interval is allowed to close (see Fig. 2-14). The subcutaneous tissue and skin are closed as the surgeon prefers. Use of a drain is optional.

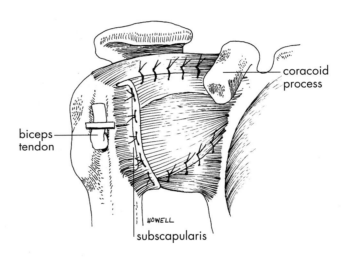

FIGURE 3-54

POSTOPERATIVE CARE (SEE CHAPTER 11)

This is a complex problem, requiring complex surgery and significant postoperative immobilization. We have used 8 weeks immobilization postoperatively, depending on the predominant direction of instability, with an obvious emphasis on holding the humeral head up against the undersurface of the acromion. The program then follows as in the classical inferior capsular shift.

Following immobilization in a sling for 3 weeks, an active rehabilitation program is started. Phase I is not performed because of the need to eliminate stretching exercises from the program. The modification of the phase is such that only active motion is used, initially limited for the first month to 90° of elevation, 30° of external rotation, and internal rotation to the belt line. Postoperative stiffness is unusual in these patients.

After 1 month without a sling, resisted exercises, emphasizing eccentric and concentric rotational strengthening, and scapular and anterior deltoid strengthening exercises are performed. Occasionally, transition between the active and resisted programs can be bridged with isometric exercises, progressing to resisted rubber tubing or Sport Cord. During this phase, the active motion can be increased to 120° of elevation, 45° of external rotation, and internal rotation to L1.

The emphasis in the program is active and strengthening exercises within a limited range, being careful not to stretch or stress the shoulder, particularly in an inferior direction.

At 1 year, there should be slight limitation of all motions and a stronger shoulder, providing functional stability.

Inferior Capsular Shift from Posterior Approach
GENERAL CONSIDERATIONS

The inferior capsular shift from the posterior approach, in our experience, has a high incidence of failure, but it has been used for multidirectional instability with predominantly inferior posterior element. Our preference in such circumstances would give consideration to approaching this problem anteriorly. The problem posteriorly relates to the deficient capsular tissue and the fleshy fibers of the infraspinatus used for this reconstruction.

Indications

The indication for a posterior shift is for multidirectional instability when predominantly posterior and inferior instability is present.

Contraindications

Contraindications would include other forms of instability.

Expectations

The expectations following inferior capsular shift from the back are guarded because there is a high incidence of failure. It would be unlikely for these individuals to return to aggressive sporting activities, although they could regain a functional shoulder with an adequate range of motion.

SURGICAL TECHNIQUE
Approach

The patient can be in the prone position (see Fig. 2-3) or, more reasonably, in the lateral decubitus position (see Fig. 2-4). A vertical posterior incision from the posterolateral corner of the acromion to the axilla is used (see Fig. 2-40), exposing the posterior deltoid (see Fig. 2-41). The deltoid is split in the direction of its fibers, much like the anterior deltopectoral approach without the guidance of the cephalic vein (see Fig. 2-42).

Procedure

The infraspinatus and teres minor are identified deep and at right angles to the deltoid fibers. The infraspinatus is incised at right angles approximately 1 cm from its insertion on the greater tuberosity, and its tendinous fibers are skived off from the underlying capsule. Some of the teres minor is left intact to protect the axillary nerve (Fig. 3-55). An incision is made in the capsule in the same direction, extending about 2.5 cm and parallel to the glenoid. At the mid portion of this flap, a right angle incision is made in the capsule, extending down to the level of the posterior labrum and glenoid (Fig. 3-56). The inferior limb is developed and stripped off the humeral neck, beginning posteriorly and, as the arm is internally rotated, mobilizing inferiorly and anteriorly (Fig. 3-57).

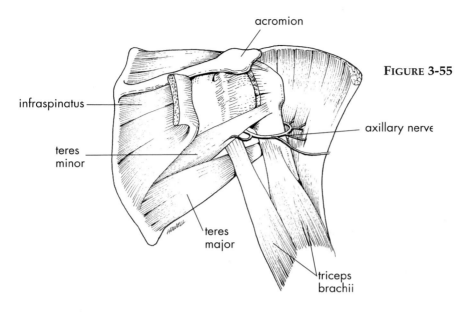

acromion

infraspinatus

teres minor

teres major

axillary nerve

triceps brachii

FIGURE 3-55

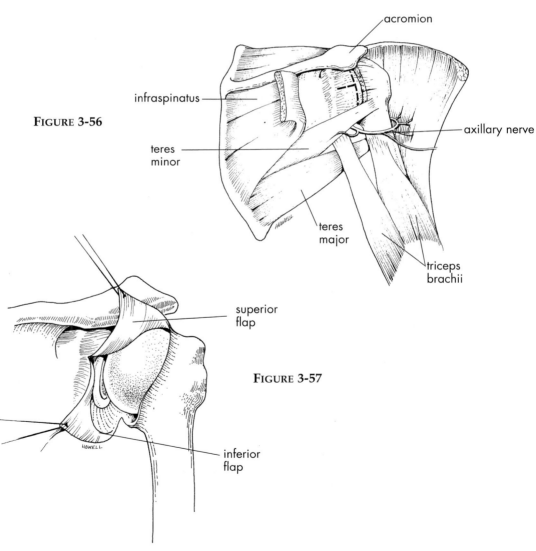

FIGURE 3-56

acromion

infraspinatus

teres minor

teres major

axillary nerve

triceps brachii

superior flap

inferior flap

FIGURE 3-57

The neck is burred (Fig. 3-58). Stripping continues, and the inferior flap is advanced superiorly and slightly laterally with the flap sutured either to a trough in the bone or to the soft tissue of the infraspinatus and the capsular cuff (Fig. 3-59). The superior flap is then overlapped inferiorly and sutured to soft tissue (Fig. 3-60). Sutures can be placed in a north-south fashion at the adjacent level of the glenoid if further cruciate reconstruction is required. The infraspinatus is then reattached from where it was taken down or may be overlapped if further stability is desired (Fig. 3-61).

Closure

The deltoid muscle is allowed to fall back together (see Fig. 2-41). Subcutaneous tissue and skin are closed as the surgeon prefers. Use of a drain is optional, but usually unnecessary.

POSTOPERATIVE CARE (SEE CHAPTER 11)

Following this procedure, the arm should be immobilized with the upper arm slightly posterior to the coronal plane and the forearm in approximately 10° to 15° of external rotation. Immobilization is required for 8 weeks following this procedure because there is a tendency toward poor tissue quality. Following immobilization, the emphasis is on strengthening rather than stretching exercises. Complete rehabilitation often requires up to 1 year. If there is some limitation of motion at that time, it might prove beneficial in avoidance of provocative positions.

Repairs for Posterior Instability
GENERAL CONSIDERATIONS

Usually the patient with posterior instability can demonstrate the instability, either by voluntary muscular contraction or by arm positioning. The diagnosis of posterior instability in those who cannot demonstrate it depends on history and physical examination features of reproduction of the symptom complex with posterior translation of the humeral head in the socket in the awake patient. During exam under anesthesia, patients with posterior instabilty occasionally do not have the excessive translation that one would expect for this instability pattern. Although the instability may be unidirectional, one must rule out a multidirectional component by examining for an excessive and symptomatic sulcus sign.

Indications

These posterior procedures are indicated for unidirectional posterior instability only.

Expectations

Historically, procedures to stabilize posterior instability have had a high incidence of failure caused by poor tissue or poor technical procedures, which are often performed in the presence of multidirectional instability. The disability associated with posterior instability is often not great, and therefore surgery is seldom indicated. In the athletic population, however, it can be a disability. Recently, the literature has suggested improved success rates, probably because of better patient selection and better attention to appropriate surgical technique and to applying appropriate tissues for reconstruction.

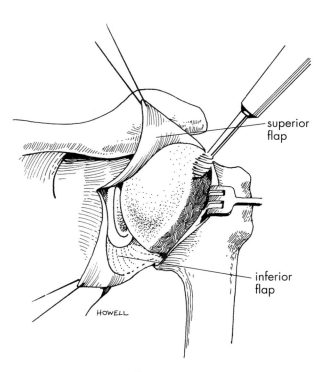

FIGURE 3-58

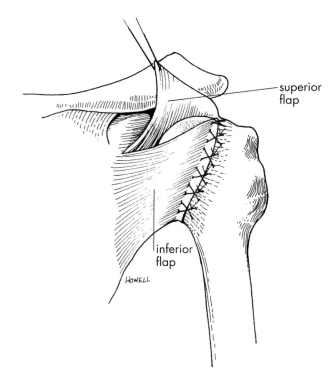

FIGURE 3-59

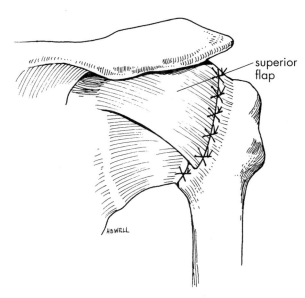

FIGURE 3-60

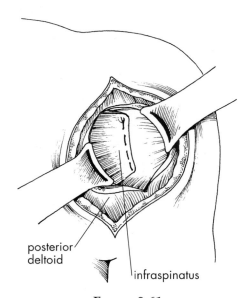

FIGURE 3-61

POSTERIOR APPROACHES
Posterior Infraspinatus Capsular Tenodesis
GENERAL CONSIDERATIONS

We have used this procedure for several years with the emphasis on suturing the tendinous portion of infraspinatus with its underlying capsule to the posterior glenoid labrum. As dissection proceeds toward the tendinous insertion on the tuberosity, the tendinous and capsular structures are noticeably thicker. Repairs with incisions more medial in the infraspinatus and capsular fibers lead to a higher incidence of failure because of the fleshy nature of the infraspinatus fibers and the paper-thin capsule.

Indications

The indications for this procedure are for symptomatic, unidirectional posterior instability.

Contraindications

Contraindications may include the presence of multidirectional instability and obvious, anterior instability. We question whether the procedure is applicable to the patient with posterior and inferior multidirectional instability.

Expectations

The success rate following posterior stabilization with this technique is approximately 85% in our present series. However, these results still do not approach those of reconstruction for routine anterior instability. Return to normal functional activities and often athletics can be expected in most cases. Patients with a traumatic etiology have a better outlook than patients with an atraumatic etiology. Those with a component of multidirectional instability do not fare as well as those with only unidirectional posterior instability.

SURGICAL TECHNIQUE
Positioning

The patient may be placed in a prone position (see Fig. 2-3) or, more appropriately, in the lateral decubitus position (see Fig. 2-4).

Approach

The skin incision posteriorly is as described under posterior surgical approaches— a straight line incision extending from the posterolateral corner of the acromion to the axilla (see Fig. 2-40), exposing the underlying deltoid (see Fig. 2-41). The deltoid is split in the direction of its fibers, and the underlying infraspinatus teres minor and greater tuberosity are identified (see Fig. 2-42).

Procedure

After the arm is positioned in roughly neutral rotation, the infraspinatus is incised at right angles to its fibers approximately at and parallel with the glenoid rim (Fig. 3-62). This incision is extended through the capsule to identify the glenohumeral joint (Fig. 3-63). This incision extends a vertical distance of approximately 2.5 cm. The posterior glenoid labrum is identified and examined and is almost always intact (Fig. 3-64). The rare situation of a labral defect (that is, reverse Bankart) will require repair with sutures to the posterior rim through drill holes or using an anchor system. This is seldom necessary, and if the glenoid

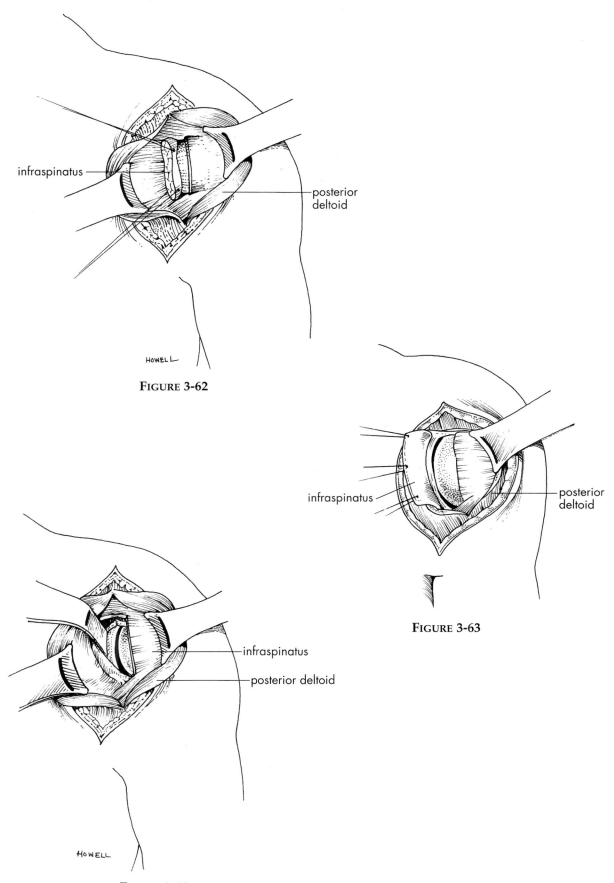

infraspinatus

posterior deltoid

HOWELL

FIGURE 3-62

infraspinatus

posterior deltoid

FIGURE 3-63

infraspinatus

posterior deltoid

HOWELL

FIGURE 3-64

labrum is of good substance, the lateral flap of the infraspinatus and the capsule are secured to the posterior glenoid labrum, holding the arm in slight external rotation (Fig. 3-65). The axillary illustration shows suturing of the infraspinatus and the capsule to post–glenoid labrum. The infraspinatus that has been incised can now be overlapped, but because of its fleshy quality, it does not add much to the repair (see Fig. 3-62). At this point, the arm should come to lie in approximately 15° to 20° of internal rotation (Fig. 3-66).

Closure

The deltoid is allowed to fall together (see Fig. 2-41), and the subcutaneous tissue and skin are closed as the surgeon prefers. The use of a drain is usually unnecessary.

POSTOPERATIVE CARE (SEE CHAPTER 11)

Because these patients have a tendency to be somewhat like multidirectional patients with questionable collagenous tissue and because there has been such a high failure rate, we recommend postoperative immobilization for 6 weeks with the upper arm slightly posterior to the coronal plane and the forearm in slight external rotation, perhaps 10° to 15°. If the instability is traumatic, 4 weeks immobilization may be appropriate.

Following removal of the immobilization device, Phase I can be implemented for approximately 2 weeks, followed by Phase II for an additional 2 weeks, followed by Phase III, while continuing to stretch the shoulder.

Posterior Glenoid Osteotomy
GENERAL CONSIDERATIONS

Posterior glenoid osteotomy has been used for unidirectional posterior shoulder instability with reasonable success. The concern regarding a posterior glenoid osteotomy relates to potential complications. The pitfalls are several. If there is a tendency toward multidirectional instability, a change in the orientation of the glenoid may cause the patient to dislocate or sublux in the opposite direction. It has never been shown that an abnormal glenoid version contributes to posterior instability and thus the rationale for changing a version is questionable. The osteotomy cut can transect the glenoid neck, causing a free-floating fragment that is difficult to secure. The osteotomy cut could be too short and, with levering into the glenohumeral joint, result in a glenoid fracture. A fracture can result in the rapid onset of glenohumeral osteoarthritis, which is a very unfortunate complication, particularly in a young patient.

Indications

The indication is unidirectional posterior instability that is symptomatic enough to warrant surgery.

Contraindications

This procedure is contraindicated in the presence of multidirectional instability.

Expectations

The failure rate is fairly high and the complication rate is of concern. But if the procedure is successful, it should produce a functional, stable shoulder.

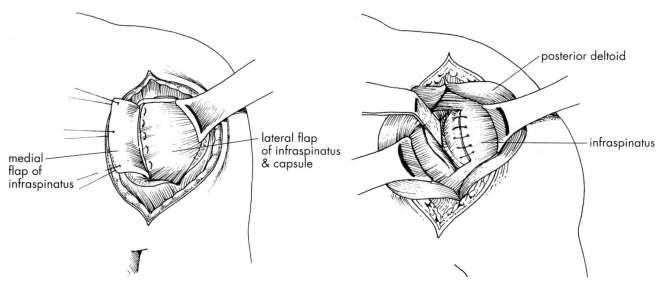

medial flap of infraspinatus

lateral flap of infraspinatus & capsule

posterior deltoid

infraspinatus

FIGURE 3-65

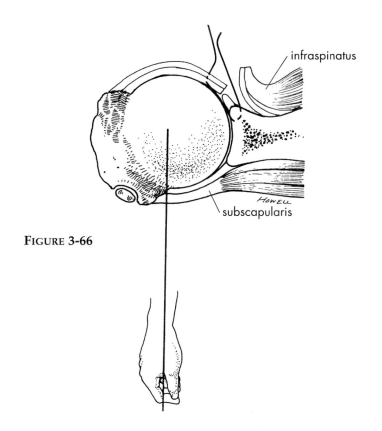

infraspinatus

subscapularis

FIGURE 3-66

SURGICAL TECHNIQUE
Positioning

For posterior shoulder instability, the patient can be placed in the prone position (see Fig. 2-3) or lateral position (see Fig. 2-4). The lateral position is preferred to allow easier control of the arm for appropriate positioning.

Approach

The approach is a vertical incision extending from the lateral corner of the acromion, to the axillary fold (see Fig. 2-40), exposing the underlying deltoid (see Fig. 3-41). The underlying deltoid is identified and spread in the direction of its fibers, midway between the acromion and the axilla. The fascia of the infraspinatus is identified, revealing the infraspinatus fibers, which run at right angles to the deltoid (Fig. 3-67, also see Fig. 2-42).

Procedure

With finger dissection, the deltoid is separated from the infraspinatus and a retractor is passed under the acromion to retract the superior aspect of the deltoid. A large retractor is placed inferiorly to retract the inferior portion of the deltoid (Fig. 3-67). An incision is made through the infraspinatus and the capsule into the joint to carefully identify the articular surface of the glenoid as it relates to the subsequent osteotomy (see Fig. 3-64). Alternatively, the infraspinatus and the teres minor can be spread apart and the underlying capsule can be incised (see Fig. 2-43). A small incision is made in the horizontal plane over the periosteum of the lateral superior angle of the acromion in the superior aspect of the wound. The periosteum is dissected off the acromion, and a triangular bone graft is excised from the posterolateral corner of the acromion, measuring approximately 1.5 to 2 cm at the base of the triangle and 1 cm from the base of the triangle to its apex (Fig. 3-68). The glenoid neck is identified approximately 1 cm from the glenoid surface. Drill holes placed in line at the osteotomy will help avoid complications (Fig. 3-69). With an oscillating saw, an osteotomy cut is made from the superior to the inferior neck of the glenoid, 1 cm from the glenoid surface, taking extreme caution to go exactly parallel with the glenoid surface (Fig. 3-70).

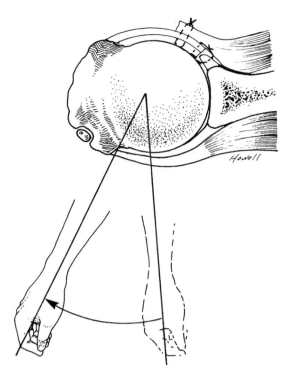

FIGURE 3-67

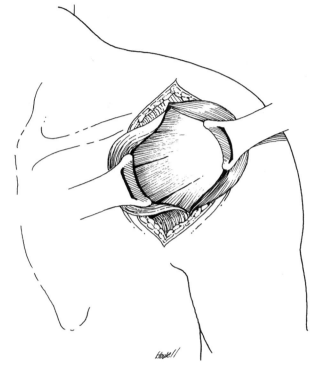

FIGURE 3-68

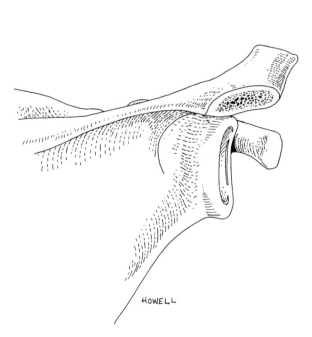

FIGURE 3-69

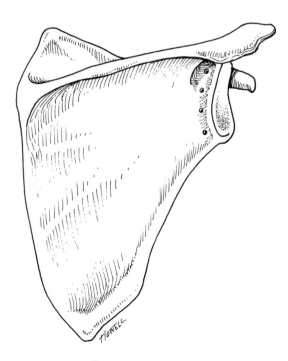

FIGURE 3-70

When it is estimated that the cut is almost through to the opposite cortex, osteotomes can be used to gently lever the osteotomy cut open as one approaches the opposite cortex (Figs. 3-71 and 3-72). Do not transgress the opposite cortex, but simply wedge open the osteotomy cut, hinging on the anterior cortex (Fig. 3-73). Too aggressive a cut will create a floating glenoid neck, which can be very difficult to secure (Fig. 3-74). Making the osteotomy cut too short poses a danger of fracture into the joint, leading to the potential devastating complications of osteoarthritis (Fig. 3-75).

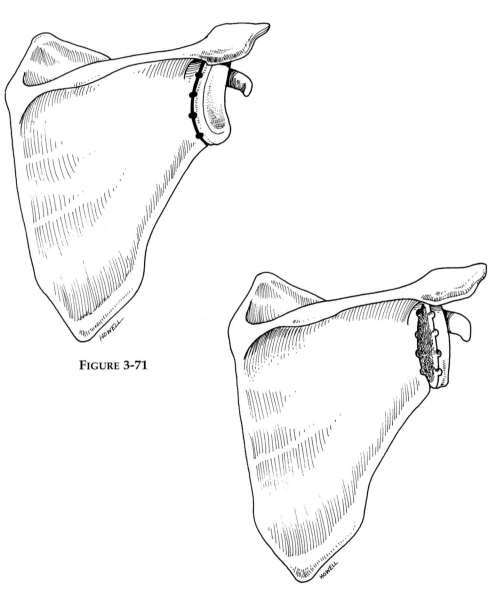

FIGURE 3-71

FIGURE 3-72

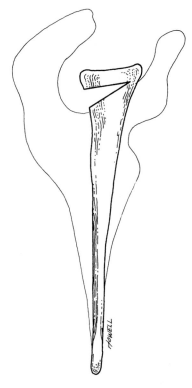

FIGURE 3-73

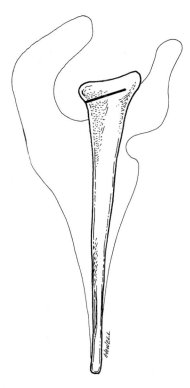

FIGURE 3-74

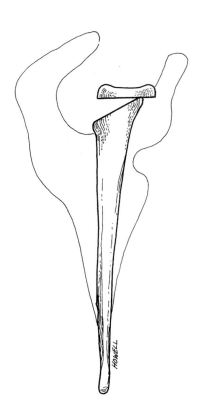

FIGURE 3-75

With osteotomes gently inserted and levered, the osteotomy cut is wedged open posteriorly and the graft is inserted (Figs. 3-76 to 3-78). A capsulorrhaphy can be performed, as can an overlapping of the infraspinatus, if desired (Fig. 3-79).

Closure

The deltoid is simply allowed to fall together, and the subcutaneous tissue and skin are closed in the usual fashion. A drain is optional at the discretion of the surgeon.

POSTOPERATIVE CARE (SEE CHAPTER 11)

Pressure dressing is applied immediately postoperatively. Fashioning the spica preoperatively allows its application in the operating room. Alternatively, an orthosis can be applied or an abduction pillow can be used to support the arm until a cast can be applied postoperatively. The shoulder should be immobilized for 3 to 4 weeks, with the upper part of the arm slightly posterior to the coronal plane and the forearm in 15° of external rotation, with enough abduction to allow hygienic care of the axilla.

After removal of the shoulder spica, passive exercises can begin, followed in 2 weeks by Phase II active exercises with terminal stretching. Approximately 1 month later, resisted exercises can be implemented along with the ongoing stretching program. The overall rehabilitation program is longer for posterior than for anterior instability, and return to normal sporting and heavy labor activities is forbidden for 6 months.

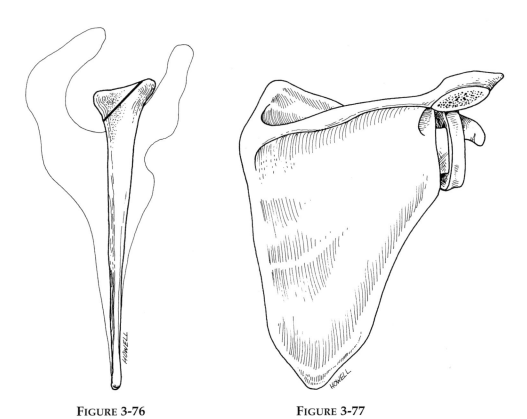

FIGURE 3-76   **FIGURE 3-77**

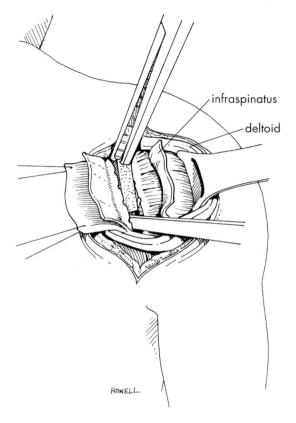

infraspinatus

deltoid

HOWELL

FIGURE 3-78

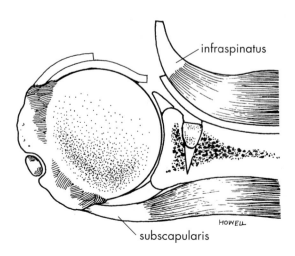

infraspinatus

subscapularis

HOWELL

FIGURE 3-79

LOCKED DISLOCATIONS

GENERAL CONSIDERATIONS

Locked dislocations of the shoulder are rare, but they must be recognized early, to provide an opportunity for the most effective treatment. A locked posterior dislocation is almost always associated with an impression defect into the lesser tuberosity. It is frequently associated with seizures, motor vehicle accidents, electrical shock, or patients with multiple traumas. Diagnosis in late cases reveals marked limitation of external rotation. An axillary view confirms the locked dislocation with an impression defect. Anterior dislocations are also often associated with seizures, particularly as a result of alcoholism, motor vehicle accidents, and multiple trauma. Impression defects are rarely associated with these lesions. They often occur in older patients and may be associated with a rotator cuff tear, which complicates reconstruction.

Locked Anterior Dislocation

GENERAL CONSIDERATIONS

A functional range of motion may often be obtained with a locked anterior dislocation if it remains unrecognized for a long time. These injuries can be diagnosed acutely, but historically the diagnosis has been missed and the patient is diagnosed late. In either case, a surgical approach is usually indicated in the active patient.

Indications

The indication for reconstruction is a functionally disabled and/or painful shoulder with an associated locked anterior dislocation.

Contraindications

The procedure is probably contraindicated in uncooperative patients such as alcoholics, especially if they have a functional range of motion without much pain.

Expectations

The expectations following reconstruction are guarded because it is a complex reconstruction that sometimes requires rotator cuff repair, reduction of the glenohumeral joint, and soft tissue balancing to maintain reduction.

SURGICAL TECHNIQUE
Positioning

The patient may be placed in the "beach chair" position (see Fig. 2-1), a semi-sitting position (see Fig. 2-2), or, more advantageously, the lateral decubitus position (see Fig. 2-3). It is sometimes necessary to approach the shoulder both anteriorly and posteriorly to obtain appropriate tissue releases and reduction of the humeral head into the glenoid fossa. Reconstruction may be necessary to keep the humeral head reduced.

Approach

The initial approach is anterior through the usual deltopectoral approach (see Fig. 2-9). Because exposure is important, an axillary approach would probably not be indicated unless the surgeon prefers this approach (see Figs. 2-10 and 2-11).

Procedure

The dislocated humeral head is identified, and the subscapularis is incised approximately 1 cm from the biceps tendon and parallel with it (see Fig. 2-17). Adequate soft tissue releases superiorly and inferiorly must be performed to allow reduction of the humeral head. If there is scar tissue in the glenoid fossa, it may require resection before reduction can be obtained. If the rotator cuff is deficient, it requires mobilization and reconstruction as described in the section on rotator cuff repair. Once the humeral head is reduced and the arm is positioned in internal rotation, the subscapularis and the capsule require reconstruction with advancement to obliterate the anterior pouch (see Fig. 3-32).

Closure

The deltopectoral interval is allowed to close (see Fig. 2-14), and the subcutaneous tissue and skin are closed in the usual fashion. Use of a drain is optional, but not usually required.

POSTOPERATIVE CARE (SEE CHAPTER 11)

Postoperative care consists of immobilization with the arm across the chest for 2 or 3 weeks, followed by range of motion exercises to regain both motion and strength on a gradual basis. The result could be a stiff stable shoulder.

When Phase I is started at approximately 2 weeks, stretching is implemented with careful monitoring of external rotation so that it does not become too limited. At 4 weeks, active exercises are begun with terminal stretching. At 6 to 8 weeks, resisted exercises are undertaken, while continuing the stretching program.

Locked Posterior Dislocations
GENERAL CONSIDERATIONS

Chronic posterior dislocations almost always have an associated impression defect of variable size. The determination of operative procedure is based on the duration of the dislocation and the size of the impression defect or, more critically, the amount of remaining articular cartilage to function in the glenoid fossa. As a result of loss of cartilage nutrition, dislocations that have been present for more than 1 year often require arthroplasty, regardless of size of the impression defect. Dislocations of less than 1 year and with a 40% or lower impression defect can be reduced and reconstructed by inserting the subscapularis into the impression defect (McLaughlin) or by inserting the subscapularis with a segment of lesser tuberosity into the defect (Neer's modification).

Indications

The indication for operating on a locked posterior dislocation is a functional disability with or without the presence of pain in a locked posterior dislocation in an active patient.

Contraindications

The procedure is contraindicated in an uncooperative patient who is susceptible to seizure or alcoholism.

Expectations

The expectations following reconstruction depend on the operative procedure. If McLaughlin's or Neer's modifications can be performed, the outcome is excellent with a functional range of painless motion. The expectation following arthroplasty is less successful in terms of range of motion, although reasonably good pain relief is possible.

SURGICAL TECHNIQUE—SUBSCAPULARIS TRANSFER (MCLAUGHLIN OR NEER MODIFICATION)
Positioning

The patient is placed in the "beach chair" (see Fig. 2-1) or semi-sitting position (see Fig. 2-2). An inflatable cuff may be placed under the ipsilateral shoulder.

Approach

An anterior deltopectoral approach is used (see Fig. 2-9). An axillary incision may be considered (see Figs. 2-10 and 2-11). The biceps tendon and subscapularis are identified (see Fig. 2-16).

Procedure

The humeral head sits posteriorly, and sometimes the anterior edge of the glenoid can be palpated. A longitudinal 3- to 4-cm incision is made adjacent to the biceps tendon into the lesser tuberosity (Fig. 3-80). An osteotome to try to elevate the lesser tuberosity with the attached subscapularis is helpful for subsequent bone-to-bone union into the defect (Fig. 3-81). It is not always possible to osteotomize a portion of bone with lesser tuberosity as described by Neer. The surgeon is often left with the option of only a soft tissue procedure as described by McLaughlin (Fig. 3-82). As the subscapularis is elevated, eventually the joint is entered and the glenoid is identified. Part of the humeral head can be visualized, and part of it is obscured by the impression defect.

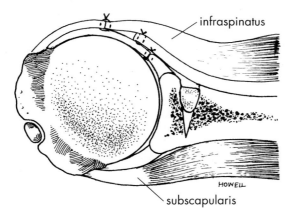

infraspinatus

subscapularis

FIGURE 3-80

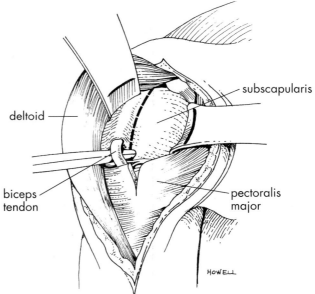

deltoid

subscapularis

biceps
tendon

pectoralis
major

FIGURE 3-81

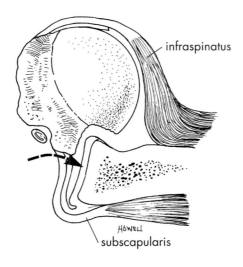

infraspinatus

subscapularis

FIGURE 3-82

Adequate tissue releases are performed superiorly and inferiorly until the humeral head can be manipulated into the joint by using an instrument such as a Bristow elevator. This instrument is used to lever into the impression defect, pushing and pulling laterally until the arm can be distracted from the locked posterior position and externally rotated to deliver the articular surface into the glenoid (Fig. 3-83). At this point, the size of the impression defect and the amount of remaining articular surface is determined, and the quality of the articular surface is assessed (Fig. 3-84). Usually at this point, rotation of the arm will reveal whether, in fact, there is going to be a functional range of motion. If the impression defect is less than 40% of the articular surface, transfer can be undertaken. The defect is denuded of scar tissue down to bleeding bone (Fig. 3-85), and cancellous screws are secured through the tendon and attached bone into the defect (Figs. 3-86 and 3-87).

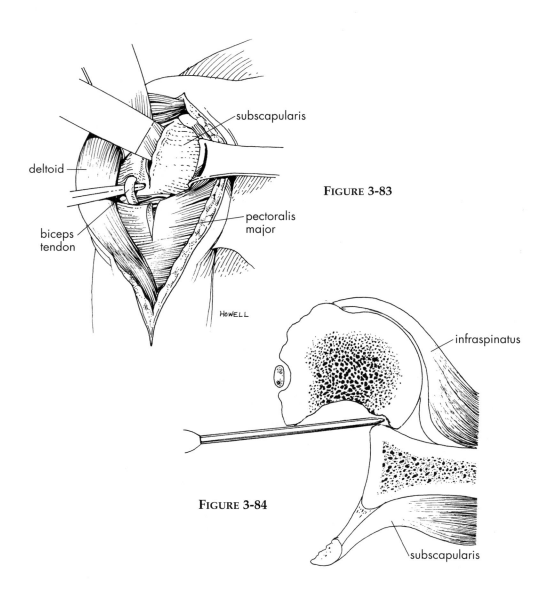

FIGURE 3-83

FIGURE 3-84

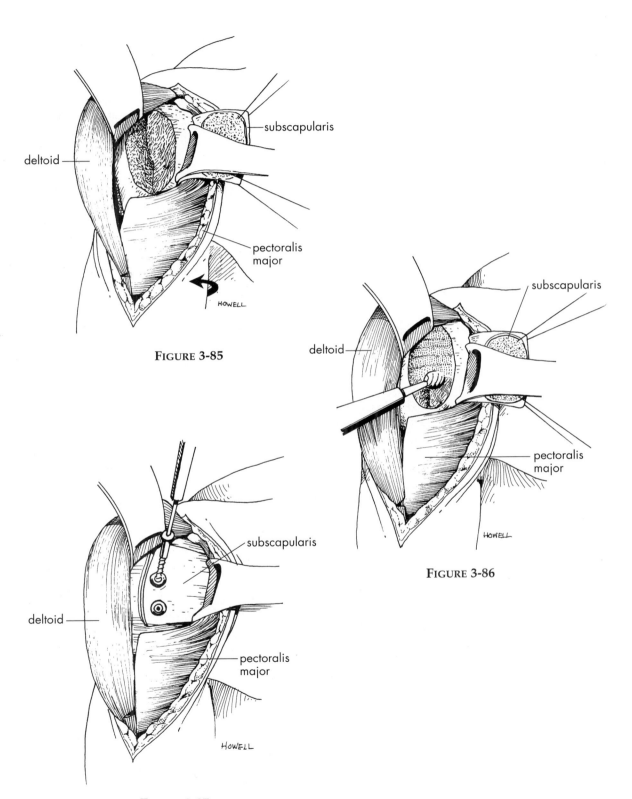

FIGURE 3-85

FIGURE 3-86

FIGURE 3-87

If there is not enough bone, drill holes can be made and sutures passed from tendon through the holes to secure the tendon into the impression defect (Fig. 3-88). Stability and rotation can then be assessed.

Closure

The deltopectoral interval is allowed to close (see Fig. 2-14). Subcutaneous tissue and skin are closed as the surgeon prefers. The use of a drain is optional, but usually unnecessary.

POSTOPERATIVE CARE (SEE CHAPTER 11)

Postoperative care is controversial. In the past, the arm was immobilized, with the forearm in slight external rotation for 4 to 6 weeks. Gradually, progressive Phase I, II, and III exercises were started. If secure fixation is obtained, particularly with screws, gentle range of motion exercises can begin initially until the subscapularis tendon is healed to the defect. At that time, active exercises can be started. Internal rotation may be limited at the beginning to prevent disrupting the repair.

SURGICAL TECHNIQUE—ARTHROPLASTY FOR LOCKED POSTERIOR DISLOCATION
Indications

The indication for arthroplasty for locked posterior dislocation is in an active patient who is symptomatic in the presence of a nonviable head, regardless of the size of the impression defect, or if the impression defect is larger than 50%, regardless of time.

The technique of arthroplasty is as described in Chapter 5 with the variation that the longer the duration of dislocation, the less retroversion should be used. For example, if the dislocation has been present for less than 3 months with a fairly large impression defect, retroversion of the humeral component should be approximately 20° rather than the usual 35° to 40°. If this dislocation had been present for 1 year with a large defect, neutral version may be more appropriate. The only other modification would be that sometimes the posterior pouch can be closed in a purse-string fashion after the head is osteotomized to lessen the tendency toward posterior subluxation.

Expectations

The postoperative expectations are less optimal than in normal arthroplasties because of the long-standing humeral head deformity in the shoulder with the tendency toward posterior subluxation. Inappropriate version or an ongoing posterior deficiency may lead to posterior instability or subluxation.

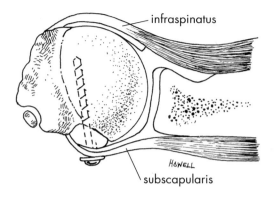

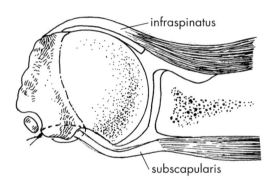

FIGURE 3-88

Rotator Cuff

4

Introduction

Tears of the rotator cuff and impingement tendinitis represent two of the most common disorders of the shoulder. Although often dealt with as separate entities, most rotator cuff tears represent an end stage of the impingement continuum. Impingement tendinitis is by definition a mechanical irritation of the rotator cuff by one or more of the various components of the acromial arch: the acromion, the acromioclavicular joint, the coracoacromial ligament, and, rarely, the coracoid process. In addition to rotator cuff damage, there may be involvement of the tendon of the long head of the biceps and the subacromial bursa. These patients complain of an aching discomfort, often associated with overhead activities and frequently accompanied by night pain. There may be a history of trauma, more often of overuse.

Physical signs vary according to the level of disease involving the rotator cuff. Patients with intact rotator cuffs, but with impingement tendinitis, will have impingement signs (Neer, Hawkins) and a painful arc at 60° to 120° of abduction. As the level of disease of the rotator cuff increases, there is a progression from tendinitis to fibrosis, to partial thickness tears, and, finally, to full thickness rotator cuff tears that increase in size with time. As the level of rotator cuff involvement increases, the physical examination picture changes. Patients with rotator cuff tears will manifest the findings of impingement tendinitis as well as muscle wasting, weakness of elevation and external rotation, and crepitus. A large tear will prohibit the patient from holding the arm in an elevated position.

It is appropriate to consider decompression acromioplasty for individuals with impingement tendinitis for whom conservative treatment fails. Care must be taken to rule out associated pathology of either the acromioclavicular joint, the rotator cuff itself, or the biceps tendon. In addition, individuals with instability problems may manifest concomitant findings of impingement tendinitis. Acromioplasty alone in these patients may be unsuccessful.

The decision-making process regarding operative treatment in these patients may be a difficult one. Several avenues of surgical treatment exist for these patients according to their level of disease. In patients with pure impingement tendinitis and an intact rotator cuff, an arthroscopic or an open acromioplasty will be adequate. In patients with Stage II disease, with small or partial thickness rotator cuffs and coexistent impingement tendinitis, the options increase. The dilemma of dealing with partial thickness remains. Is decompression alone adequate, and at what degree of partial tear (that is, 75%) should decompression be accompanied by some form of reconstruction? An arthroscopic acromioplasty followed by a miniarthrotomy to repair the rotator cuff may be an option. Preoperative planning is crucial to define the status and size of the rotator cuff tear. As the pathology increases and the size of the tear grows, most surgeons lean toward a formal open repair. With massive tears, the surgeon must often consider debridement alone, sometimes with acromioplasty performed either by open or by arthroscopic means. All of these techniques require thorough preoperative evaluation, including physical examination, and preoperative testing, including arthrogram, magnetic resonance imaging, or both. Magnetic resonance imaging allows staging of the disease regarding tear size. Whichever procedure is used, meticulous care of the deltoid and an adequate decompression are necessary to ensure success in the treatment of rotator cuff problems. With massive tears, a high-riding humeral head and a thin acromion may suggest debridement without acromioplasty.

To properly treat rotator cuff pathology, one must understand the various sizes and types of rotator cuff tears. Tears are usually classified according to location, size, and extent of involvement. Full thickness tears are broken down into small (less than 1 cm), involving the supraspinatus (Fig. 4-1, *A*); medium (1 to 3 cm), involving the supraspinatus (Fig. 4-1, *B*); large (3 to 5 cm), involving the supraspinatus and infraspinatus (Fig. 4-1, *C*); and massive (greater than 5 cm), involving the supraspinatus, infraspinatus, and subscapularis (Fig. 4-1, *D*).

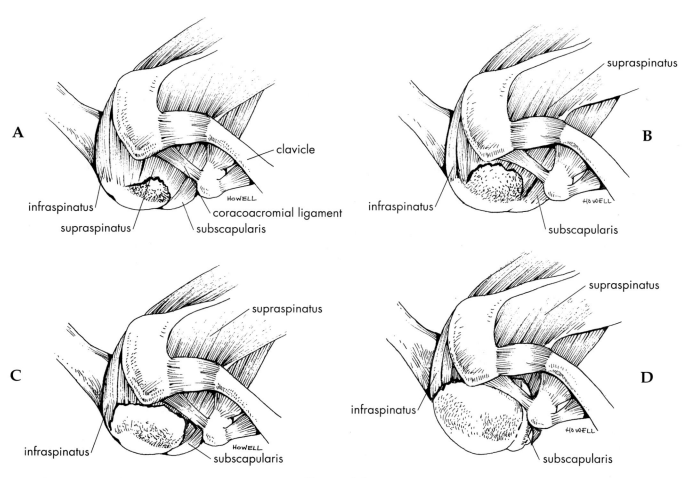

FIGURE 4-1

The configuration of the size may vary from L-shaped to oval to triangular. Interval tears may also be present, each requiring a different method of mobilization and repair. Almost all tears, however, start at the greater tuberosity, progress medially (some posteriorly) and then anteriorly, with one of the eventual configurations. Mobilization is directed toward closing the interval lesions and eventually reapproximation to a trough at the level of the old anatomical neck (Fig. 4-2). Partial thickness tears are classified according to location relative to the joint. There are bursal tears (Fig. 4-3, *A*), intraarticular tears (Fig. 4-3, *B*), and interstitial (Fig. 4-3, *C*) or midsubstance partial thickness rotator cuff tears.

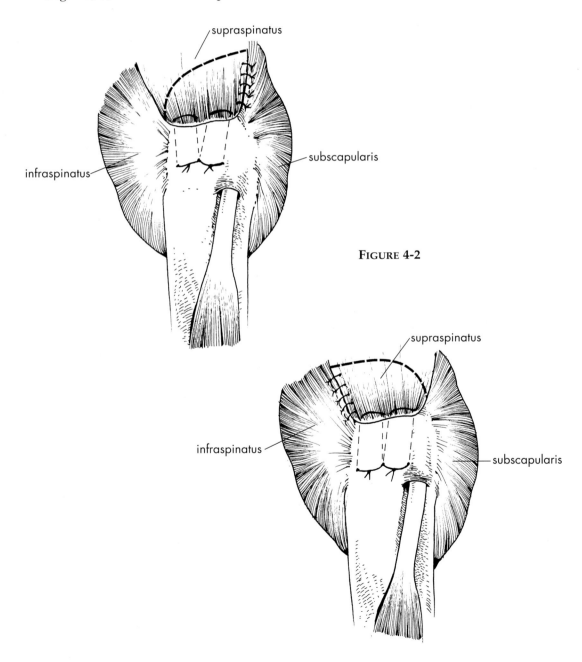

FIGURE 4-2

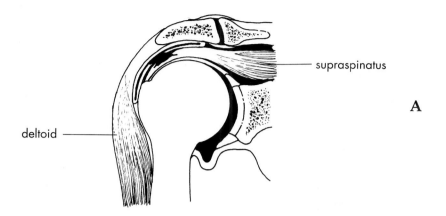

supraspinatus

deltoid

A

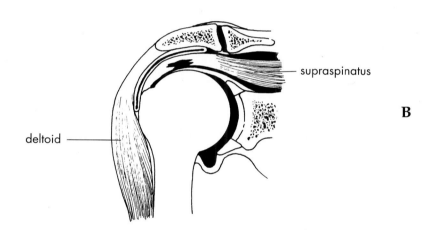

supraspinatus

deltoid

B

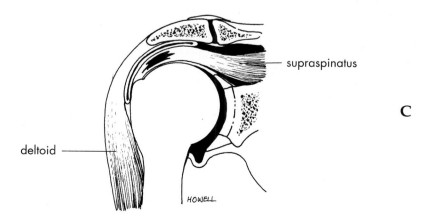

supraspinatus

deltoid

C

HOWELL

FIGURE 4-3

Acromial morphology, as described by Morrison and Bigliani, consists of three types: Type I is flat (Fig. 4-4, *A*), Type II has a gentle concavity (Fig. 4-4, *B*), and Type III is hooked (Fig. 4-4, *C*). Various studies have shown the relationship between the hooked Type III acromion and coexistent rotator cuff tears. When one considers an arthroscopic acromioplasty in patients with impingement, the outlet view helps to define not only acromial morphology in terms of the anteroinferior prominence but also helps to demonstrate the relative thickness of the acromion and the amount that should be arthroscopically resected.

Acromioplasty
GENERAL CONSIDERATIONS

An acromioplasty, whether done arthroscopically or open, must in all cases adequately decompress the involved structures. Attention should be given not only to the acromion but also to the acromioclavicular joint, the coracoacromial ligament, and, in rare cases, the coracoid process. The presence of associated rotator cuff tears or biceps pathology must be treated accordingly. The arthroscopic approach is described in detail in Chapter 10.

Indications

An acromioplasty is appropriate only after an adequate trial of conservative measures, including nonsteroidal anti-inflammatories, physical therapy, and judicious use of injections. Patients failing those measures with continued physical findings of impingement tendinitis (such as a positive impingement sign and impingement test), night pain, and preservation of motion are candidates for operative treatment. An adequate trial of nonoperative management might continue for a minimum of 6 months.

Contraindications

Contraindications include a primary problem of instability. These patients must be carefully evaluated and the instability treated first. A relative contraindication is adhesive capsulitis. Attempts should be made to resolve the adhesive capsulitis before performing an acromioplasty, since in many of these patients their symptoms of tendinitis are attributable to the limited motion and capsular irritation and not to impingement.

Expectations

Of those patients undergoing open acromioplasty who meet the appropriate criteria, 80% to 90% will have improvement in pain and return to a functional shoulder. Failure with this procedure is usually the result of either an inadequate decompression or an error in diagnosis. The prognosis of returning a high profile thrower to pre-injury level is guarded.

SURGICAL TECHNIQUE
Positioning

The patient is placed in the "beach chair" position (see Fig. 2-1) or in the semi-sitting position (see Fig. 2-2). A half-liter IV bag or inflatable cuff is placed beneath the involved scapula, and the head is secured with either a headrest or light taping (see Fig. 2-1). Impervious drapes are applied to block out both the axilla and the head, and the arm is prepped and draped free.

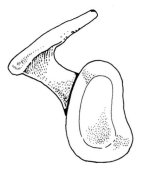

A

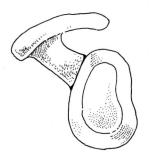

B

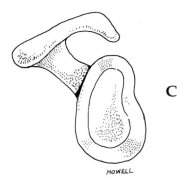

C

HOWELL

FIGURE 4-4

Approach

Two approaches exist to the exposure of the anterior acromion and subacromial space: deltoid on (see Fig. 2-34) and deltoid off (see Fig. 2-32). In both situations, a superolateral approach is used as described in Chapter 2. The skin incision may vary (Fig. 4-5). Our preference is an incision perpendicular to Langer's lines (Fig. 4-5, *a*). This skin incision provides an excellent cosmetic result, is in line with any necessary deltoid split, and thus facilitates retraction of the various layers without compromising exposure. Fig. 2-31 illustrates these skin incisions. The incision shown in Fig. 2-31, *b* allows the deltoid to be split in the direction of the skin.

In the deltoid off approach, with the skin incision completed, the deltoid is identified and incised off the anterior acromion (see Fig. 2-32). Using electrocautery, the surgeon makes an incision through the fascia down to the anterior acromial bone. The incision begins at the anterolateral corner of the acromion and courses medially to the anteromedial corner of the acromion, identified by the acromioclavicular joint. This incision is based 0.5 cm back from the anterior aspect of the acromion. In cases of significant anterior acromial spurring or ossification of the coracoacromial ligament, the surgeon may use the anterior aspect of the acromioclavicular joint as a guide to determine the true anterior margin of the acromion. As will be shown in the rotator cuff section, this incision may then be extended laterally and distally in the raphe between the middle and the anterior deltoid (see Fig. 2-33). This is only helpful for cuff reconstruction. After the deltoid is released off the anterior acromion, the subacromial space and the coracoacromial ligament as it inserts on the undersurface of the acromion are readily visualized.

The deltoid on approach uses a longitudinal incision beginning 2 cm posterior to the anterior aspect of the acromion, coursing anterolaterally in line with the deltoid fibers over the anterior aspect of the acromion (Fig. 4-6). This technique uses a subperiosteal dissection of the aponeurotic tissue of the deltoid dissected off the anterior and superior surface of the acromion. This detached cuff of deltoid and fascia is designed for subsequent reattachment at the completion of the procedure. The deltoid is split in the direction of its fibers up over the acromion, elevating it subperiosteally so that it may later be repaired side-to-side. The incision extends into the deltoid muscle in the direction of its fibers to create an elliptical split, allowing side-to-side closure. One third of the length of the incision is up on the acromion and two thirds below the anterior border of the acromion. It is important to dissect the fascia off the anterior acromion even with the inferiorly attached fascia. With the subacromial space and anterior acromion exposed, the coracoacromial ligament is seen attaching to the undersurface of the acromion. In this illustration, the acromioplasty cut is outlined from above with the underlying cuff intact. Fig. 4-7 shows the same view with an underlying cuff tear.

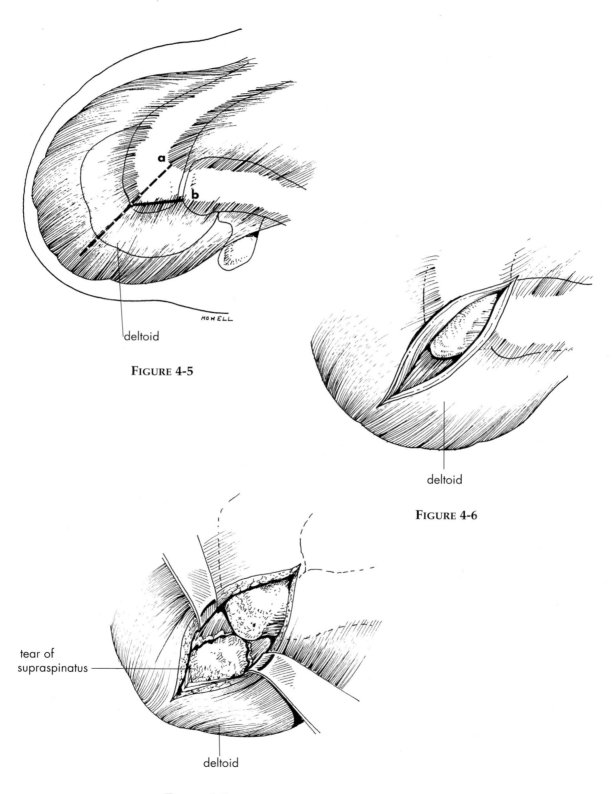

deltoid

FIGURE 4-5

deltoid

FIGURE 4-6

tear of
supraspinatus

deltoid

FIGURE 4-7

Procedure

With the acromion exposed, an anteroinferior decompression acromioplasty is performed, using either an osteotome or an oscillating saw. A Darach retractor is placed beneath the acromion to protect the underlying rotator cuff (Fig. 4-8). The intent of the acromioplasty is to resect only the anteroinferior prominence of the acromion (Fig. 4-9). If the cut is too vertical, an inadequate decompression may result (Fig. 4-10); if it is too horizontal, the cut may be carried back to the neck of the acromion, creating an acromial fracture (Fig. 4-11). Examination of the undersurface of the acromion in preoperative films will allow one to appropriately triangulate the cut by aiming for the apex of the undersurface of the acromion, a distance of approximately 1.5 cm posterior to the anterior margin. This triangulation of the cut will create a gentle transition and appropriate decompression of the subacromial space, creating a Type I, or flat, acromion (Fig. 4-9).

The acromial bone is grasped with a Kocher clamp, and the coracoacromial ligament is sectioned (Fig. 4-12). The acromial branch of the thoracoacromial artery may be encountered at this stage and require coagulation.

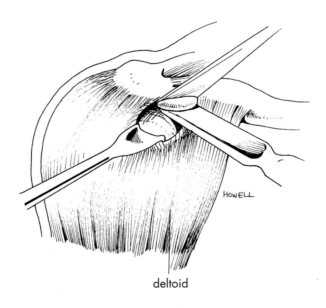

deltoid

FIGURE 4-8

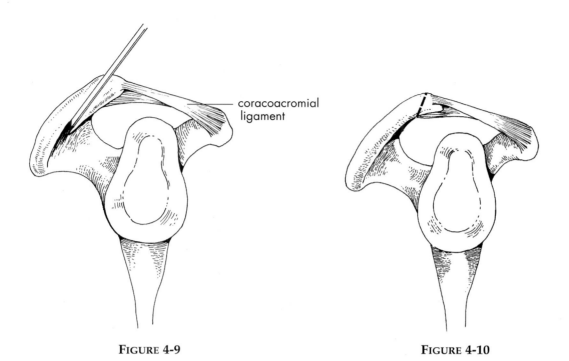

coracoacromial
ligament

FIGURE 4-9

FIGURE 4-10

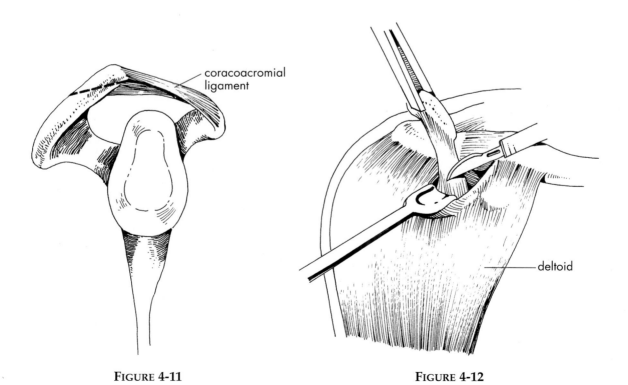

coracoacromial
ligament

FIGURE 4-11

deltoid

FIGURE 4-12

The rotator cuff is then inspected. If excessive bursal formation obscures adequate visualization, it can be excised. The undersurface of the acromion and acromioclavicular joint should be palpated and any irregularities or osteophytes excised to adequately decompress the entire subacromial space medially (Fig. 4-13). This can be done with an osteotome, file, burr, or a combination of these. In cases of painful acromioclavicular joint arthritis, a concomitant arthroplasty may occasionally be performed (Fig. 4-14).

Closure

Once decompression of the cuff is complete and its integrity is confirmed, the wound is irrigated and closure begun. With the deltoid on approach, the deltoid is repaired side-to-side with the first suture at the anterior acromion (Fig. 4-15). In similar fashion, the deltoid off approach brings the anterior deltoid, both superficial and deep fascial layers, back to the anterior acromion. With this approach, a suture is passed through both fascial layers and, if necessary, through the anterior acromial bone. Drill holes may be necessary in the osteotomized acromion for secure closure (Fig. 4-16). If the deltoid has been split distally for exposure, it is reapproximated distally.

POSTOPERATIVE CARE (SEE CHAPTER 11)

Passive range of motion exercises may be started as soon as the day of surgery, especially in situations in which regional anesthesia (scalene blocks) was used. With long-acting blocks, it is optional to start the patient on a continuous passive motion machine in the recovery room. Even with general anesthesia, we begin immediate range of motion exercises. These passive exercises are continued for the first week or until pain lessens and motion increases to allow active motion and terminal stretching. Strengthening resistive exercises are started at approximately 2 to 4 weeks. Both deltoid approaches are usually reapproximated securely enough to allow early active motion, usually within 1 to 2 weeks, or sooner if pain permits.

Adequate healing of the soft tissues and return of strength requires approximately 3 months. At this time, return to manual labor, athletic endeavors, or both may be considered.

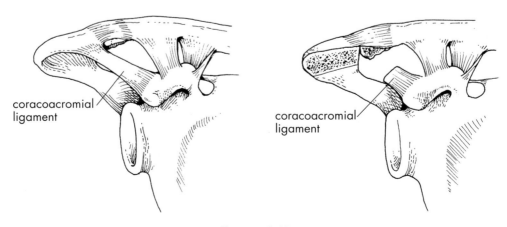

coracoacromial ligament

coracoacromial ligament

FIGURE 4-13

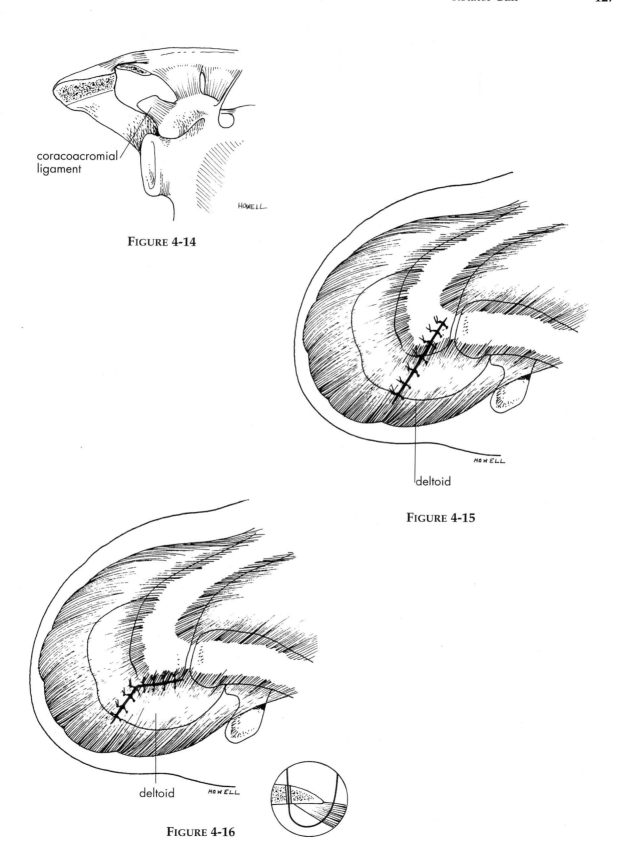

coracoacromial
ligament

HOWELL

FIGURE 4-14

deltoid

HOWELL

FIGURE 4-15

deltoid

HOWELL

FIGURE 4-16

Rotator Cuff Repairs
GENERAL CONSIDERATIONS

Rotator cuff surgery represents a sizable undertaking for both the patient and the surgeon. Depending on the size of the tear and the patient's age, rehabilitation may be recommended. Thus, it is important that the surgeon have an appreciation for the patient's needs, expectations, and level of disability, as well as an idea of the anticipated pathology. Is it a small simple tear, a large tear, or is there evidence of a massive, irreparable tear? Is there cuff arthropathy, acromioclavicular joint disease, or biceps attrition? All of these questions must be asked and answered, either preoperatively or, in some cases, intraoperatively. A careful history and physical examination combined with the judicious use of arthrography and magnetic resonance imaging will provide enough information to determine cuff size and repairability preoperatively. Magnetic resonance imaging, reliably performed and interpreted, is the best method to stage the disease process, especially related to size of tear.

Indications

Active patients with pain, diminished active range of motion, decreased strength, and a confirmed full thickness rotator cuff tear are ideal candidates for surgery. Patients with partial thickness tears are also amenable to operative intervention. For most surgeons, pain is the main indication for surgery in either partial or full thickness tears. Preoperative staging through magnetic resonance imaging, arthroscopic inspection, or both will help demonstrate the relative thickness of a partial tear. In patients with a greater than 50% involvement of the rotator cuff tendon, we elliptically excise that portion of the pathology and repair either side-to-side or, more often, to a bony trough. The injection of methylene blue with concentration in the area of a partial thickness tear may indicate significant involvement suggesting greater than 50% tearing. It is often difficult to preoperatively stage the disease with the use of the arthroscope. Intraarticular tears are easily determined, but intrasubstance tears are obviously impossible to determine. Bursal side tears are sometimes difficult to stage because of extensive scarring.

Contraindications

Relative contraindications in rotator cuff surgery include severely limited passive motion (adhesive capsulitis), which should be addressed before formal cuff surgery, severe medical disability, minimal functional demands, or limited pain. Coexistent glenohumeral arthritis may necessitate a concomitant hemiarthroplasty at the time of potential cuff repair. In this situation, hemiarthroplasty alone may be performed if the cuff tear is too large to repair.

Expectations

With cuff repair, 80% to 90% of patients should achieve pain-free function of the shoulder above the horizontal. Patients with massive, irreparable rotator cuff tears will often obtain pain relief with little improvement in strength and motion with debridement and decompression alone. In those individuals with compromised tissue and larger tears, a limited goals program should be suggested. This is done to provide the patient with appropriate expectations. Recent studies indicate that large and massive tears, although repaired at the time of surgery, may come apart. These patients often continue to have pain relief, but functional weakness.

SURGICAL TECHNIQUE

Position

The patient is placed in the "beach chair" position. A half liter bag or inflatable cuff is placed under the involved scapula, and the head is secured with either a headrest or light taping (see Fig. 2-1). Impervious drapes are applied to block out both the axilla and the head, and the arm is prepped and draped free. The semi-sitting position is preferred by some surgeons (see Fig. 2-2). Even the lateral position can be used (see Fig. 2-4) if it is combined with arthroscopy in the lateral position (see Fig. 2-5).

Approach

Rotator cuff surgery begins with an incision similar to that used for the open acromioplasty procedure (see Fig. 4-5). One may use either the deltoid on (see Fig. 4-6) or deltoid off (see Fig. 4-8) approach. In both cases, the deltoid is detached subperiosteally and then split longitudinally in line with its fibers (see Fig. 2-33). In most cases, a tag suture is placed at the most inferior extent of the deltoid. The deltoid is split to avoid retraction of the deep fascial layers and further separation. Before beginning the rotator cuff repair, the decompression acromioplasty is performed, resecting the anteroinferior margins of the acromion (see Figs. 4-8, 4-9 and 4-12). Similarly, any inferior osteophytes at the acromioclavicular joint are excised (see Fig. 4-13), and if indicated, occasionally an acromioclavicular arthroplasty (see Fig. 4-14) is performed, excising the lateral 1.5 cm of the clavicle.

Procedure

With the decompression completed, the rotator cuff tear is more readily visualized (Fig. 4-17; also see Fig. 4-7). If bursal tissue obscures the tear, some of it may be excised, keeping in mind that this tissue provides cells to aid in subsequent healing. The extent of the tear is defined, the margins of the retracted tendon are identified, and horizontal tag sutures are placed to facilitate mobilization (Fig. 4-18). Simple vertical sutures placed anteromedial, and one posteromedial, are usually sufficient. These sutures may be incorporated in a later repair. The ideal suture for repair is probably a strong, nonabsorbable, braided polyester suture. Christian Gerber suggests a No. 3 suture is best (unavailable in North America). We use a special-order 1 mm Deknatel suture.

The sutures are placed in a horizontal fashion so that the margins of the tear are free from any suture material. This placement allows the surgeon to trim any necrotic or degenerative portions of the cuff tear without compromising the traction stitches. Regardless of how large the cuff tear is at initial inspection, the surgeon should be willing to spend most of the operative time on mobilization. Traction sutures are placed in the supraspinatus medially, the infraspinatus posteriorly, and, if need be, the subscapularis anteriorly. As few sutures as possible will avoid confusion. Grouping these traction sutures according to the tendon in which they are placed will help at the time of repair.

With traction applied to the sutures, digital dissection in the subacromial space is used to free all residual adhesions along with any adhesions between the deltoid and the rotator cuff (Fig. 4-19). In all tears, the coracohumeral ligament, as it attaches near the subscapularis/supraspinatus interval, may be identified and released (Fig. 4-20). This release is taken to the level of the coracoid process, being careful not to violate the rotator cuff interval itself.

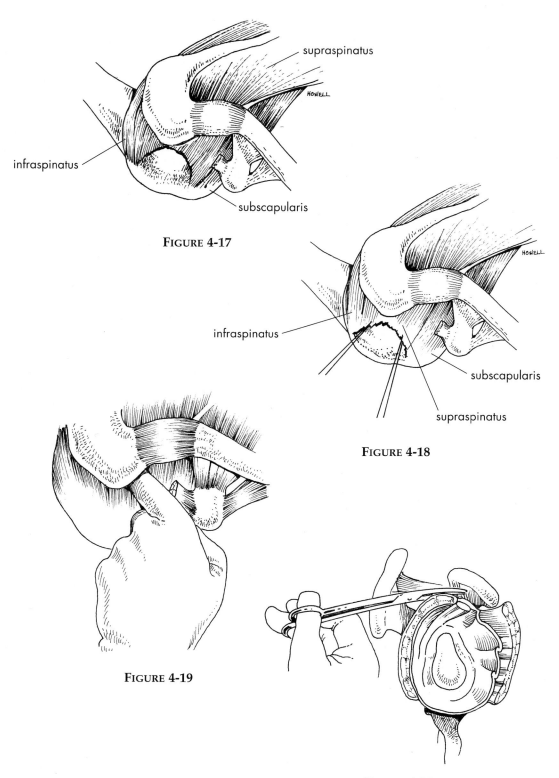

supraspinatus

infraspinatus

subscapularis

Figure 4-17

infraspinatus

subscapularis

supraspinatus

Figure 4-18

Figure 4-19

Figure 4-20

Some larger tears will demonstrate marked retraction and pericapsular adhesions. A helpful technique to assist with mobilization is an intraarticular release at the capsulolabral junction. The capsule is released off the scapular neck outside the labrum, thus leaving the labrum intact (Fig. 4-21). This release is extended along the neck of the glenoid for approximately 1 cm. To visualize the interior of the joint and the undersurface of the cuff, we use a lamina spreader placed beneath the anterior aspect of the acromion and against the humeral head. This step allows distraction of the humeral head and adequate visualization of the undersurface of the cuff. The release of the capsule from the labrum begins posteriorly on a right shoulder at the nine o'clock position and is carried around anteriorly to approximately the three o'clock position, avoiding injury to the biceps and its attachment at the superior margin of the glenoid (Fig. 4-22). Once the capsule is released, additional dissection may be carried out, but one must not be overly aggressive, especially posteriorly, because of the position of the suprascapular nerve, which lies on the posterior scapular neck.

In many rotator cuff repairs, especially in small- and medium-sized tears, a direct repair to a transverse bone trough is adequate. Fig. 4-23 shows the creation of the trough. Fig. 4-24 shows the suturing of the tendon for the trough. This procedure provides the best biomechanical construct. In large and massive tears, the orientation of the repair may require more than a simple tendon-to-bone technique. As described previously, tears will extend either posteromedially or anteromedially (see Fig. 4-2). Larger tears will typically require side-to-side tendon repair and then repair to a bone trough. In large tears, the tear is uniform in its retraction. In this situation, mobilization of the tendon all the way to its original position at the greater tuberosity is impossible.

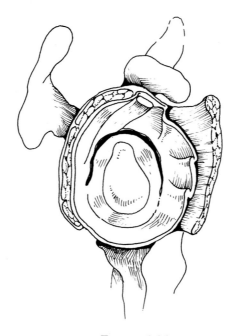

FIGURE 4-21

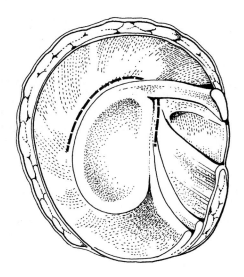

FIGURE 4-22

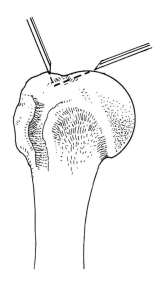

FIGURE 4-23

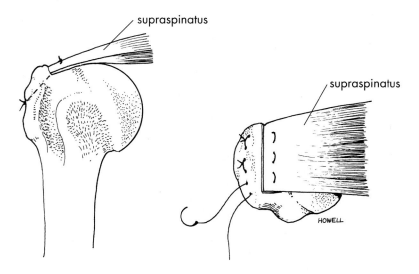

supraspinatus

supraspinatus

FIGURE 4-24

As such, the anterior and posterior margins of the tear are brought together in the center line of the tear to create an apex to the tear (Fig. 4-25). In tears in which there is a longitudinal component with medial extension, the apex of this defect is closed before placing sutures from the bone trough to the cuff. Fig. 4-25 demonstrates the use of the traction sutures in both the infraspinatus and subscapularis, drawing these two margins together to create the apex in the cuff repair. While the margins are held together, repair sutures of No. 2 nonabsorbable material are placed in a figure eight fashion, beginning medially and progressing laterally (Fig. 4-26).

The next step is the creation of a bone trough into which the lateral margin of the cuff will be repaired. This process begins with a vertical cut at or about the original insertion of the rotator cuff into the greater tuberosity (Fig. 4-23). This vertical cut determines how far the cuff must be mobilized; therefore, with larger tears one might move closer to the articular surface with this cut. One must also consider that the lateral bridge through which sutures pass is the lifeline to the repair and must be kept intact. The second cut is horizontal and begins somewhere on the articular surface to create a trough with a gentle transition from articular surface to cancellous bone with an ultimate depth of approximately 3 to 4 mm. Special instrumentation can be used to create the trough (Linvatec Rotator Cuff Instrumentation) (Fig. 4-27). Fig. 4-27, *A* initiates the hole, and Fig. 4-27, *B* completes the hole. With sutures then placed from the lateral margin of the greater tuberosity, back into the base of the trough, through tendon, and back out through the tuberosity, a smooth transition is achieved from the superior margin of the cuff to the greater tuberosity as demonstrated from the front and from above (Figs. 4-26, 4-28, and 4-29).

With the apex of the repair achieved and the bone trough created, the final step is repairing the cuff to the cancellous bed. Nonabsorbable suture material is used, and we use a suture technique that brings the suture material from lateral to the tuberosity, through the bone trough medially, from inferior through cuff, and then looped back inferiorly and brought through cuff again, exiting through the trough once again. As shown previously, this pulls the rotator cuff repair down into the bony trough, obtaining a secure repair with the smooth transition from cuff to bone (Figs. 4-28 and 4-29).

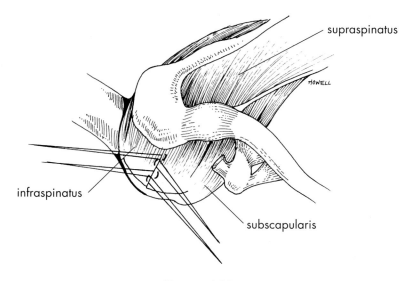

FIGURE 4-25

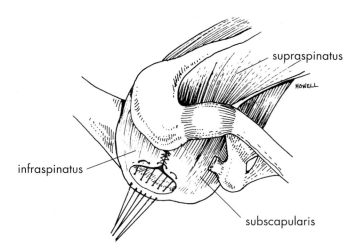

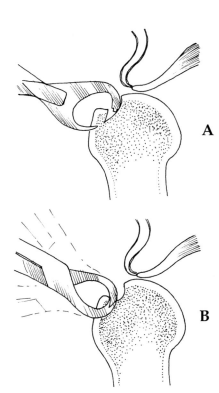

FIGURE 4-26

FIGURE 4-27

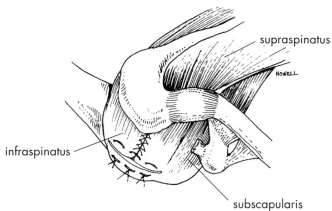

FIGURE 4-28

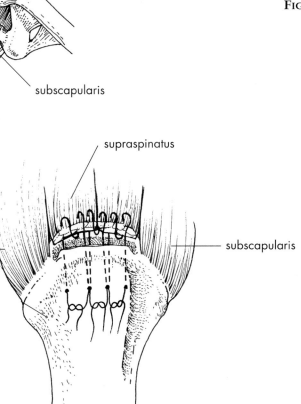

FIGURE 4-29

Many methods of suturing are used to secure the tendon to the trough. In the past, we have tied the knot on the tendon side with good success. Recently, we have used the loop suture, which is vertical, goes through the tendon twice, and secures the repair to the trough. Although some suture is interposed, this does not seem to be a problem and has worked quite well. Christian Gerber has described a Mason Allen stitch that holds well (Fig. 4-30). Fig. 4-31 shows the steps in this stitch. Fig. 4-32 shows a simple stitch, Fig. 4-33 shows a mattress stitch, and Fig. 4-34 shows a modified Kessler 2. Fig. 4-35 shows a stitch described by Steve Snyder. Rarely, some surgeons may use bone anchors (Fig. 4-36).

In the majority of cases, completion of the cuff repair will signal a time for closure. Rarely, before closure, one will encounter severe degenerative fraying of the biceps tendon as it passes through the groove and a tenodesis may be indicated. Usually, the biceps is left on its own, particularly if it is displaced medially, and usually it is unnecessary to suture it to its original trough (Fig. 4-37). A thorough inspection of the intraarticular portion of the biceps and that portion of the biceps as it exits the joint is appropriate. Should there be marked fraying of the tendon or a strong preoperative demonstration of biceps pathology, an inspection of the biceps intraoperatively is appropriate. Should the fraying be significant (greater than 50% involvement), consideration for a tenodesis may be appropriate. The biceps should be preserved if at all possible. A discussion of techniques for biceps tenodesis is located at the end of this chapter.

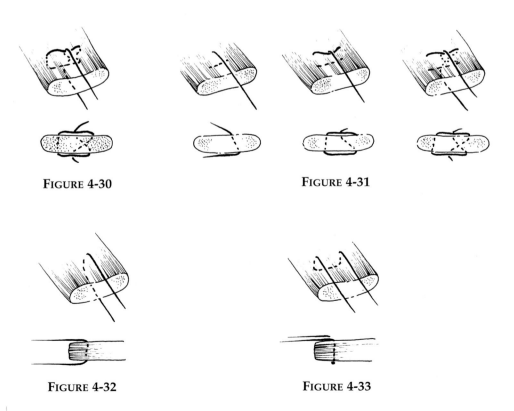

FIGURE 4-30   FIGURE 4-31

FIGURE 4-32   FIGURE 4-33

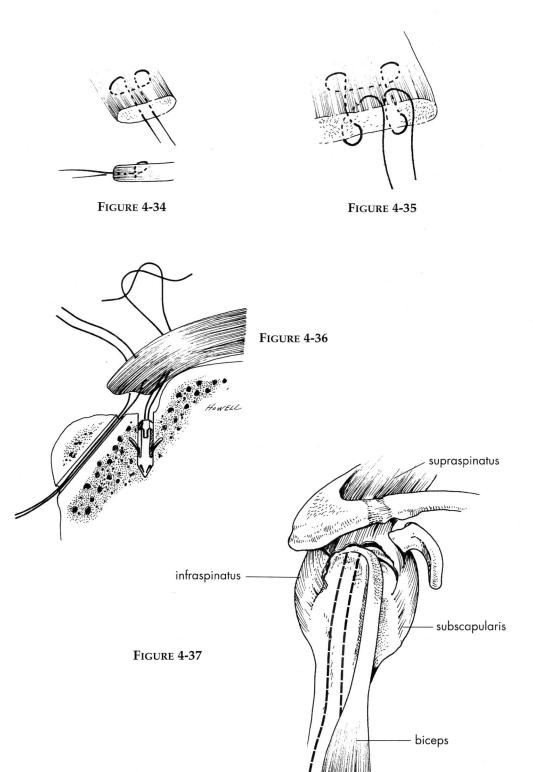

FIGURE 4-34

FIGURE 4-35

FIGURE 4-36

HoWELL

FIGURE 4-37

supraspinatus

infraspinatus

subscapularis

biceps

The keys to a successful repair are good tissue, adequate mobilization, adequate trough and bridge, secure repair to the trough with strong nonabsorbable sutures, and an appropriate suture technique.

Occasionally, the rotator cuff defect and resulting retraction will be too substantial to allow a primary repair. In such cases one may consider a subscapularis transfer (Fig. 4-38). This procedure involves a release of only the subscapularis, separate from the underlying capsule. This release begins adjacent to the lesser tuberosity and is carried vertically down to the junction of the middle and inferior third of the subscapularis. Using sharp dissection and tag sutures, the subscapularis tendon is carefully dissected free from the underlying capsule. The dissection continues medially until the muscle-capsule interval is reached. At this point, blunt dissection alone will free the subscapularis from the underlying capsule. Only the upper two thirds of the subscapularis tendon, free from capsule, is transposed and rotated superiorly (Fig. 4-39). This mobilized tendon is then secured to a trough and secured to the anterior subscapularis to close the defect (see Fig. 4-13, *B*).

If a rotator cuff repair is not achieved by conventional methods, a reasonable option is the use of the long head of the biceps as a tendon graft or suturing the ends of the tendon to the biceps (Fig. 4-40). First, the biceps is transposed 1.5 cm laterally and posteriorly to its anatomical position within the groove. A new trough is created for the tendon in this position, and it is tenodesed in that setting. At this point several options exist, the first of which is leaving the biceps attached to the glenoid intraarticularly and applying a limited number of sutures, incorporating the tendon into the rotator cuff repair. Alternatively, the biceps may be released at its insertion into the glenoid, filleted in half and opened, and used as a surface graft to bridge the repair.

With massive cuff defects that are irreparable, debridement alone is sometimes the most appropriate procedure. With a thin acromion of a very high-riding humeral head, decompression may take away the remaining fulcrum, compromising subsequent elevation of the arm. The thinner the acromion, the less decompression should be performed. In advanced situations, such as cuff arthropathy, decompression is probably not indicated.

Closure

Closure depends on whether a deltoid on or deltoid off approach was used. In the case of a deltoid off approach, closure is achieved with repair of the deltoid to the exposed anterior acromion, using nonabsorbable sutures in a figure eight fashion. Drill holes may be required in the anterior acromion to secure the deltoid and fascia to the acromion (see Fig. 4-16). With the deltoid on approach, which is elliptical, a side-to-side closure should be possible, with the first suture beginning at the level of the anterior acromion (see Fig. 4-15). The subcutaneous layer is closed in a standard fashion with a running subcuticular stitch for the skin.

The arthroscopic decompression is described in Chapter 10. The principles of the mini-open procedure are the same as for the open procedure. For this procedure, we use the deltoid on approach.

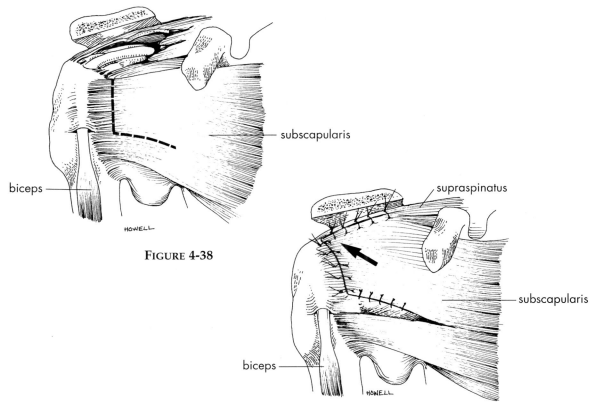

subscapularis

biceps

Figure 4-38

supraspinatus

subscapularis

biceps

Figure 4-39

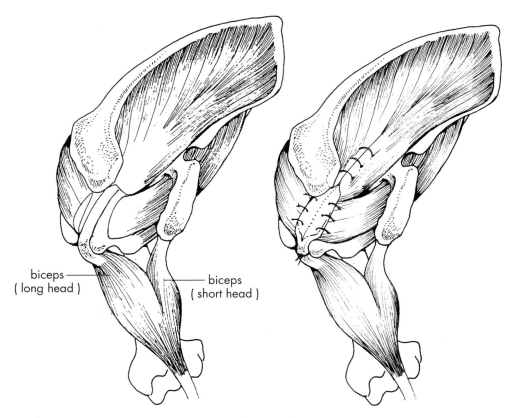

biceps
(long head)

biceps
(short head)

Figure 4-40

POSTOPERATIVE CARE (SEE CHAPTER 11)

A shoulder immobilizer is applied. In cases of large or massive tears when the repair is tenuous, an abduction pillow may also be used. The indications should be those individuals in whom the cuff repair was achieved only with the arm in a slight degree of abduction. In those cases, as the arm is brought down into an adducted position at the side of the body, the surgeon will note excessive tension at the site of the cuff repair. In such instances, using an abduction pillow for approximately 6 weeks might provide adequate time for the cuff repair to heal. During this time, initial passive exercises may be conducted above the pillow, trying not to compromise the repair.

The postoperative rehabilitation of these patients must be individualized according to the size of the tear, the quality of tissue, the tension on the repair, and the patient's personality. As a rule of thumb, rehabilitation must be tailored around the fact that it probably takes 6 to 8 weeks for tendon-to-trough healing.

In all patients, passive range of motion exercises are usually started on the day of surgery. Using an interscalene block as a regional anesthetic allows easy passive motion, particularly by a therapist, without pain. Even if a general anesthetic was used, early physiotherapy should be started. In most small and medium tears, passive range of motion exercises continue for the first 6 weeks. In large and massive tears, passive motion should be continued up to 8 weeks. Passive exercises, using the opposite extremity, consist of motion in the planes of forward elevation and external rotation. Internal rotation is delayed for 3 weeks because it stresses the repair. Abduction is avoided because of the resulting impingement and the stress of a long lever arm and because it is not a usual functional motion.

Active exercises are started once a reasonable range of passive motion has been achieved and the tendon is securely healed to the trough. The transition from a passive to an active program often involves the patient returning to the supine position, especially for elevation. Terminal stretching continues in elevation and in external and internal rotation. As the patient's strength and comfort level improve, resistive exercises are added, working on rotational and anterior deltoid exercises.

Terminal stretching and resistive exercises are started when the patient has a relatively painless range of active motion, which is usually at 3 months. Early in recovery, isometric resistive exercises below the horizontal may help tone up the muscles. As the patient's strength and motion improve, dynamic resistance is performed in rotation and in flexion for the deltoid. It often takes 6 months before the patient can lift the arm above the horizontal in comfort and confidence. Free weights and isokinetic exercises may be added under the guidance of a physical therapist. (See Chapter 11 for more information.)

Biceps Tenodesis
GENERAL CONSIDERATIONS
Isolated cases of biceps tendinitis are very uncommon. Although intrinsic attritional tears of the biceps do occur, the surgeon is cautioned to avoid missing the usual associated pathology such as tears of the rotator cuff, chronic impingement tendinitis, or acromioclavicular joint arthritis. In those rare instances of isolated recalcitrant biceps tendinitis, tenodesis may be considered. Appropriate physical examination and preoperative testing to ensure integrity of the rotator cuff and the absence of other disease are important.

Indications

The most common indication for a biceps tenodesis is biceps pathology encountered during a rotator cuff repair or proximal humeral fracture. Very rarely, one will need to do an isolated biceps tenodesis for attritional pathology alone. Occasionally, a young active individual will sustain an acute tear of the long head of the biceps. In this setting, a tenodesis is the only option. Usually, biceps tendon tears are not repaired. Occasionally, patients have late pain at the proximal belly of the tear, and these tears can be mobilized superiorly and tenodesed to eliminate the pain. Biceps tendon tenodesis can be performed at the time of rotator cuff repair.

Expectations

Patients undergoing a tenodesis with an isolated bicipital tendinitis may expect excellent return of function and relief of pain in approximately 80% of the cases. The patient should be warned that there may be an associated decrease of power in supination and elbow flexion relative to the normal contralateral side. Even in the presence of an unrepaired biceps, elbow flexion is weakened by only supination by 30%.

SURGICAL TECHNIQUE
Positioning

The patient is placed in the "beach chair" position with the arm draped free (see Fig. 2-1). Impervious drapes to block out the axilla and face are placed. A pillow may be placed under the ipsilateral shoulder to place the arm in a more advantageous position for approach.

Approach

The approach for an isolated tenodesis is a longitudinal anterior incision beginning 2 to 3 cm inferior to the anterior acromion. With the arm in 10° of internal rotation, the biceps groove is directly anterior (Fig. 4-41). The deltoid is split bluntly. The bicipital groove is exposed, and the transverse ligament is released. In some instances, arthrotomy may be preceded by arthroscopy with an arthroscopic release of the intraarticular origin of the long head of the biceps. At the same time, a spinal needle may be used to localize the exit point of the tendon from the joint, thereby localizing the arthrotomy site for subsequent tenodesis. If the biceps is ruptured and pulled out of the groove, its tendon will retract distally and be rolled up midway down the arm. Therefore, either two incisions or a long anterior incision may be required.

Procedure

With the tendon released and the groove exposed (Fig. 4-42), a high-speed burr is used to decorticate the area (Fig. 4-43). The tendon is then placed back into the trough, and one of several different techniques is used to secure it. A popular technique is a single, double-pronged, soft tissue staple that secures the tendon within the groove (Fig. 4-44). A portion of the stump is sewn back on itself with non-absorbable suture (Fig. 4-45).

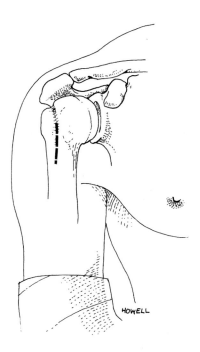

FIGURE 4-41

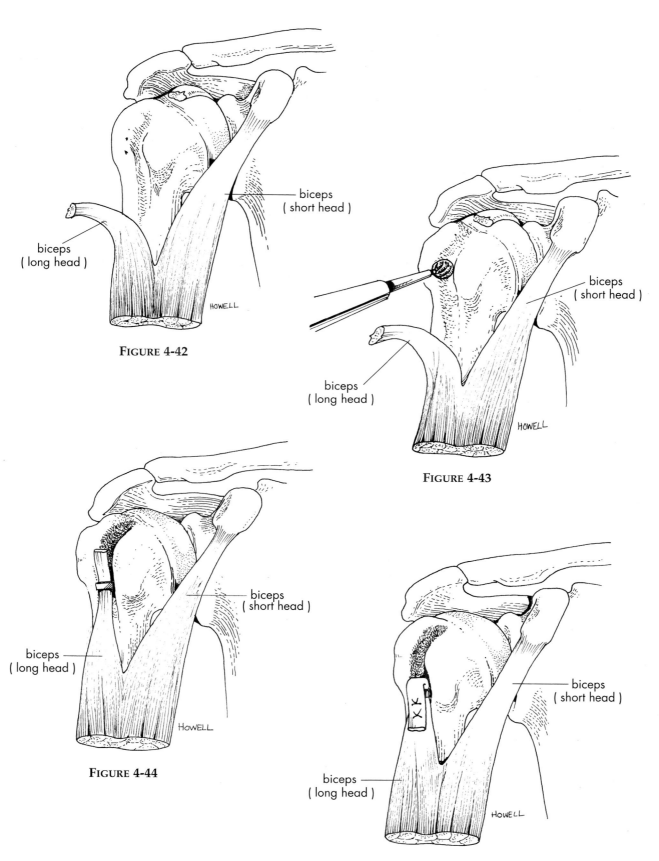

biceps
(long head)

biceps
(short head)

HOWELL

FIGURE 4-42

biceps
(short head)

biceps
(long head)

HOWELL

FIGURE 4-43

biceps
(short head)

biceps
(long head)

HOWELL

FIGURE 4-44

biceps
(short head)

biceps
(long head)

HOWELL

FIGURE 4-45

Similarly, sutures placed in a vertical mattress fashion through the cortical margins of the groove and the tendon may be used (Fig. 4-46). Another option is a bony keyhole, into which the knotted tendon is inserted (Figs. 4-47 and 4-48). With the tenodesis completed, the surgeon should palpate the superior rotator cuff to ensure integrity. Any evidence of impingement should be addressed with concomitant acromioplasty.

Closure

The deep and superficial deltoid fascial layers are reapproximated, and the subcutaneous and skin layers are closed in standard fashion. A sling is applied.

POSTOPERATIVE CARE (SEE CHAPTER 11)

Passive range of motion exercises are started on the second postoperative day for both the shoulder and the elbow. The patient is carefully instructed in the progressive extension of the elbow as pain allows. Often, full extension is not achieved until 5 or 6 weeks. The patient is further cautioned against active flexion of the elbow, which could disrupt the tenodesis. Active exercises without resistance for both the shoulder and the elbow may be started at 2 or 3 weeks. Strengthening exercises may be started at 4 to 6 weeks, with no heavy, strenuous labor or athletic endeavors attempted until 2 or 3 months.

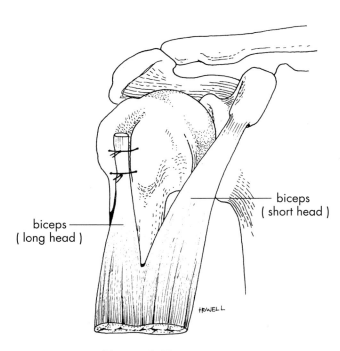

biceps (long head)

biceps (short head)

FIGURE 4-46

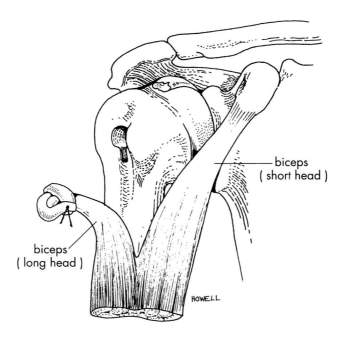

biceps
(short head)

biceps
(long head)

FIGURE 4-47

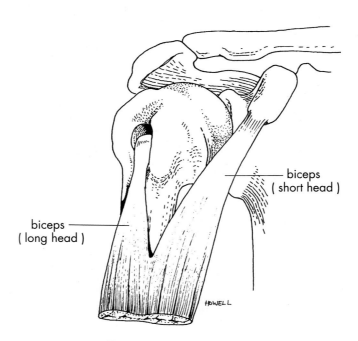

biceps
(short head)

biceps
(long head)

FIGURE 4-48

Arthrotomy for Excision of Calcium Deposits

GENERAL CONSIDERATIONS

The presence of discrete intratendinous calcium deposits is often detected during routine shoulder x-rays for other diagnoses. Occasionally, a calcium deposit will represent the isolated source of shoulder pain. These patients complain of a severe level of discomfort unrelieved by rest and unrelated to position or activity, unlike the diagnosis of rotator cuff tendinitis or tears. They will often be able to point directly to the area of the deposit, typically near the supraspinatus insertion. Most calcific deposits are located in the watershed area near the greater tuberosity in the supraspinatus tendon.

Indications

Those patients failing to respond to conservative measures, including needle aspiration, may be candidates for removal of the deposit, via either arthrotomy or arthroscopy. If there is an antecedent history of impingement, these patients should have an acromioplasty as part of their procedure. The longer the process has been present, the greater the argument for an associated acromioplasty at the time of excision. If the patient has a relatively short history of shoulder pain attributable to the calcific deposit (that is, less than 3 to 4 months) and unrelieved by conservative measures, excision of the deposit alone should be effective.

Expectations

Excellent results should be anticipated in the majority of patients with a full return of strength and motion and a resumption of work and athletic endeavors.

SURGICAL TECHNIQUE

Positioning and Approach

With the patient in a "beach chair" position, a 3- to 4-cm incision is made, beginning at the anterolateral corner of the acromion and coursing distally in line with the fibers of the deltoid (see Fig. 2-35, *a*). A transverse skin incision may be used (see Fig. 2-35, *b*). The deltoid is split bluntly, and its deep fascia is opened longitudinally (see Fig. 7-1).

Procedure

The underlying rotator cuff tendon is now readily visualized. Often, the specific location of the deposit is in question. In most cases, the area of involvement will be white with a surrounding area of hypervascularity. Perforating the suspected area with an 18-gauge needle will either reveal a gritty feel or provide a small discharge of chalky white material confirming the location (Fig. 4-49). Then, a 1- to 2-cm incision is made in the direction of the fibers of the rotator cuff, and the deposit is removed with a curette.

Closure

One or two simple stitches in a figure eight fashion of a nonabsorbable No. 2 suture material may then be used in the cuff to repair the defect, after which routine closure of deltoid (Fig. 4-50) and skin may be performed.

POSTOPERATIVE CARE (SEE CHAPTER 11)

Passive motion is begun on the first postoperative day. Active exercises are added during the next 2 weeks. Resistive exercises are begun when a comfortable full range of active motion is achieved, usually in 3 to 4 weeks. Manual labor and athletics may be resumed in 2 months.

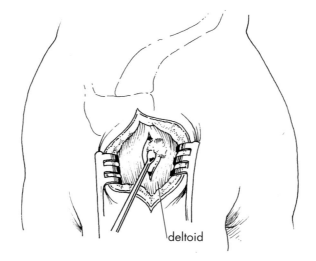

FIGURE 4-49

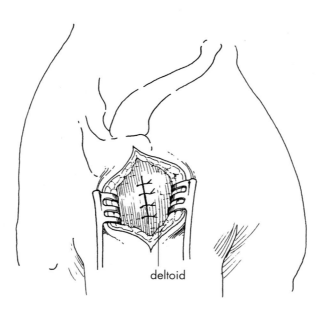

FIGURE 4-50

Arthritis

5

Introduction

Unconstrained arthroplasties have proven beneficial for arthritic conditions of the glenohumeral joint. There seems to be little indication for constrained arthroplasty systems in the shoulder because of the high failure rates. For many years, the Neer system was the standard in North America. Newer systems have become available, consisting of modular components with more variation in head sizes and glenoid configurations.

Standard operative technique involves cement fixation of the glenoid component and noncemented or press fit of the humeral component. These techniques have provided excellent results, although glenoid loosening rates have been reported with increasing frequency in long-term studies. Bony ingrowth is possible with both the humeral and glenoid components, and noncemented glenoid components are available.

Osteoarthritis, rheumatoid arthritis, and avascular necrosis are the most common pathologies requiring total shoulder arthroplasty. In general, excellent pain relief and functional improvement can be expected.

Cases in which the rotator cuff is irreparable require special consideration. Perhaps in these circumstances, hemiarthroplasty may be indicated, or occasionally the alternative application of a constrained system may be considered. Hemiarthroplasty may also be considered in cases of humeral head destruction in the absence of glenoid involvement.

Arthroplasty of the Shoulder
(Hemi versus Total Shoulder Arthroplasty)
GENERAL CONSIDERATIONS

The indications for hemi versus total shoulder arthroplasty can be confusing. In general, an intact rotator cuff with anything beyond a very mild degree of glenoid involvement would suggest the application of a total shoulder arthroplasty. Advanced cuff deficiency, such as in rheumatoid arthritis or cuff tear arthropathy, and inability to obtain reconstruction of rotator cuff, allowing a congruent glenohumeral fit, would suggest hemiarthroplasty as the best alternative. Similarly, with humeral head destruction and a normal or very minimally involved glenoid, particularly in the younger patient, hemiarthroplasty may be desirable. Hemiarthroplasty may be performed in patients with a four-part proximal humeral fracture. It may also be considered in patients with partially deficient glenoid bone stock or in situations in which reconstruction proves extremely complex.

In most circumstances, however, total shoulder arthroplasty is the procedure of choice, relying on achieving a congruent fit between humeral head and glenoid. It usually offers slightly superior pain relief compared to hemiarthroplasty.

Indications

The obvious indication for arthroplasty is a painful shoulder with glenohumeral destruction. The usual diagnoses are osteoarthritis, rheumatoid arthritis, avascular necrosis, or old fractures. There is usually associated functional disability, which by itself is rarely an indication for surgery.

Contraindications

The contraindication for total shoulder arthroplasty or hemiarthroplasty is inadequate bone stock. This procedure may also be contraindicated in active infection or in situations with significant muscle paralysis.

Expectations

The expectations regarding either hemiarthroplasty or total arthroplasty are excellent in terms of pain relief and functional improvement. The functional improvement often depends on the pathological diagnosis and the status of the proximal humerus. The prognosis is perhaps not as good in old fracture patterns requiring tuberosity osteotomies and cuff reconstruction, compared with patients with osteoarthritis and an intact rotator cuff. Patients with more advanced rheumatoid arthritis with cuff deficiency and marked glenohumeral destruction would not fare nearly as well functionally as a young patient with osteoarthritis with good muscles and intact rotator cuff. Many of these young patients return to work and sports such as golf, tennis, and skiing, especially at a recreational level.

The expectations regarding hemiarthroplasty are related to the underlying disease process. Slightly less effective pain relief can also be expected with hemiarthroplasty. Cuff arthropathy and patients with advanced rheumatoid arthritis will obviously not have as good an outcome with hemiarthroplasty in terms of functional improvement and would fall into the category of limited goals expectation.

SURGICAL TECHNIQUE
Positioning

The patient is placed in the "beach chair" position (see Fig. 2-1) or semi-sitting position (see Fig. 2-2). The glenohumeral joint must be just outside the confines of the lateral border of the operating table. This placement allows appropriate posterior retraction to access and provide exposure to the glenoid when required. An inflatable pillow can be placed under the ipsilateral shoulder. Prophylactic antibiotics and a very thorough scrub of the surgical area are extremely important in the procedure.

Approach

The surgical incision is the same, whether undertaking a hemiarthroplasty or a total shoulder arthroplasty (see Fig. 2-23). The underlying deltoid and pectoralis are revealed (see Fig. 2-24). The approach is an extended deltopectoral approach with appropriate releases of the coracoacromial ligament and the pectoralis raphe (see Fig. 2-26). Tension can be taken off the deltoid by releasing approximately 1 cm of the deltoid insertion from the humeral shaft (see Fig. 2-27). Tension can also be taken off the deltoid by abducting the arm during the surgical procedure.

Procedure
Z-plasty Lengthening

In the presence of limitation of external rotation (for example, less than 30°), particularly in osteoarthritis, a Z-plasty lengthening of the subscapularis should be considered. The subscapularis is longitudinally dissected off the underlying tuberosity at the level of and immediately adjacent to the biceps tendon, a distance of approximately 2.5 cm (Fig. 5-1, *A*). As one progresses medially, the subscapularis is teased off, and the underlying capsule is left behind. With the subscapularis retracted medially, the capsule is incised parallel with the biceps tendon. Lengthening of 1 cm equals the potential gain of 20° of external rotation. Repair of the subscapularis during closure can be overlapped (Fig. 5-1, *B*) or end-to-end (Fig. 5-1, *C*).

Usual Subscapularis Incision for Arthroplasty

In the absence of a Z-plasty lengthening, the subscapularis and capsule are incised together approximately 1 to 1.5 cm medial to the biceps tendon and parallel with it (Fig. 5-2; also see Fig. 2-28), which is at the junction of the articulating and nonarticulating surface of the humeral head (see Fig. 2-20). Adequate releases must then be performed superiorly by going up to the level of the interval and inferiorly, even stripping some of the capsule off the neck (Fig. 5-3).

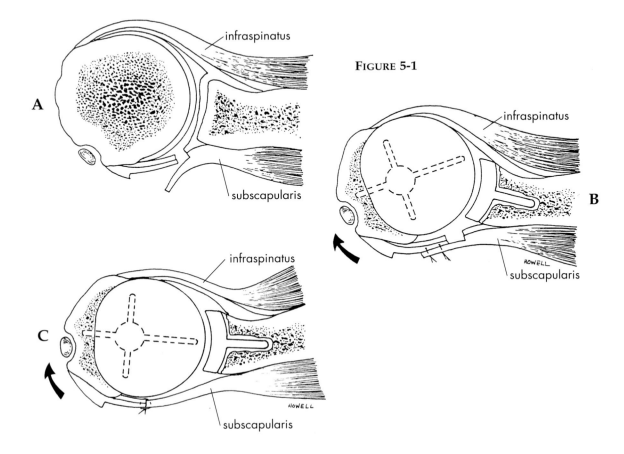

FIGURE 5-1

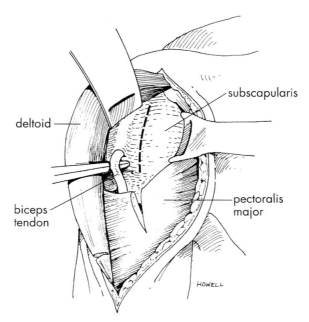

deltoid

subscapularis

biceps
tendon

pectoralis
major

HOWELL

FIGURE 5-2

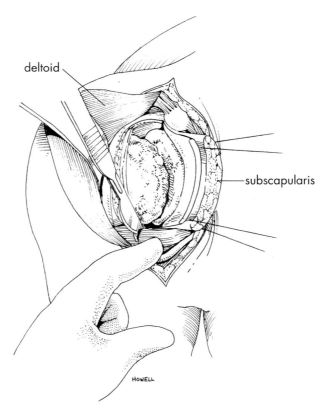

deltoid

subscapularis

HOWELL

FIGURE 5-3

Most surgeons prefer to carefully isolate, identify, and protect the axillary nerve (Fig. 5-4). With superior dissection, care must be taken not to incise the biceps. Stay sutures are positioned through the subscapularis and the capsule for retraction and subsequent ease of reattachment (Fig. 5-5). Capsular release from the glenoid is performed at the six o'clock position where the triceps resides (Fig. 5-6). With adequate releases and progressive external rotation, the humeral head is delivered into the wound. A Darrach retractor can be placed posterior to the humeral head and anterior to the glenoid to protect the glenoid and posterior structures during the osteotomy cut (Fig. 5-7).

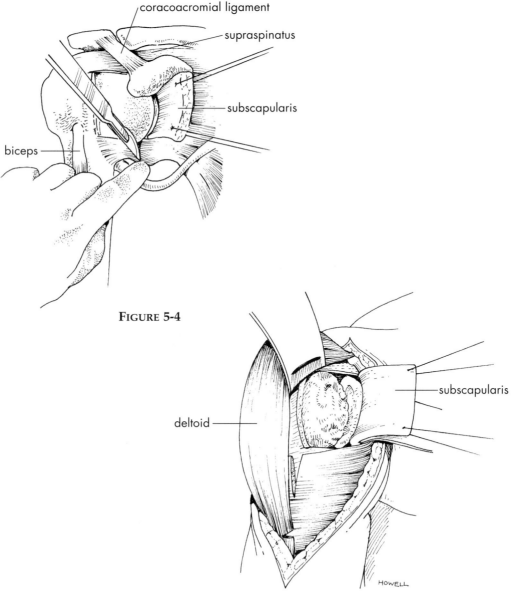

FIGURE 5-4

FIGURE 5-5

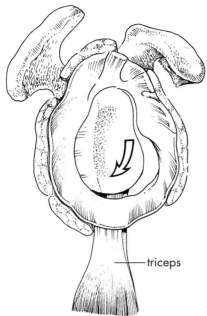

FIGURE 5-6

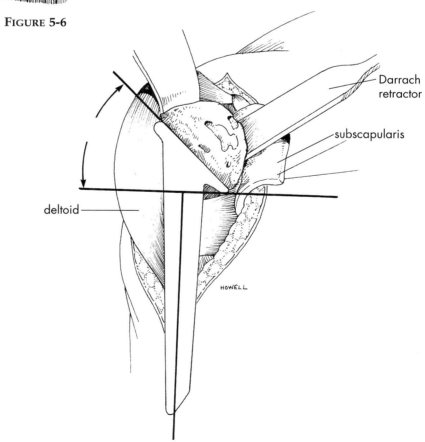

FIGURE 5-7

Depending on the arthroplasty system used, a guide may be used at this time to determine the appropriate osteotomy cut. The humeral component should sit in approximately 35° to 40° of retroversion. There are several clues in directing the osteotomy cut to achieve this end. The forearm and humerus should be externally rotated approximately 35° to 40° (Figs. 5-8 and 5-9). This rotation allows the cut to be made at right angles to the plane of the shaft and head, achieving the appropriate retroversion. Another clue is that the lateral flange should lie just posterior to the bicipital groove (7 mm). A common error is to make the osteotomy cut too vertical. If this happens, the humeral head may lie too far distally within the system, leaving a prominent greater tuberosity leading to subsequent impingement. The osteotomy cut may be performed with either an oscillating saw or an osteotome. The superior cut usually begins at the junction of the head and the greater tuberosity (Fig. 5-10). Once the cut is started and the direction is set, the arm can be further extended, adducted, and externally rotated to more easily deliver the humeral head into the wound for an easier osteotomy cut.

With completion of the osteotomy cut, the medullary canal is reamed (Fig. 5-11). Some systems (Biomet) require reaming at right angles so that the prosthesis is inserted in the appropriate retroversion. Other systems allow more flexibility with circumferential reaming. With the osteotomy cut in place, the version has been predetermined, leaving little room for variation unless the osteotomy cut is changed or there is an asymmetrical fit of the undersurface of the humeral head onto the osteotomy cut. To avoid a shaft fracture, overzealous reaming should be avoided, particularly in osteopenic bone. The canal should be reamed up to its maximum canal diameter without compromise to the cortical bone. A trial prosthesis can be inserted to assess orientation and fit (Fig. 5-12). The amount of bone resected from the head should roughly equal the size of the humeral head component to be used (Fig. 5-13). At this point, appropriate stem and head size can be selected and a decision made as to whether secure press fitting will be obtained.

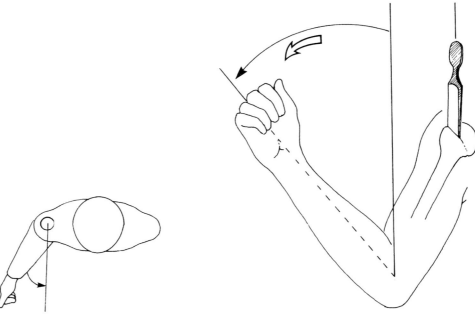

FIGURE 5-8   **FIGURE 5-9**

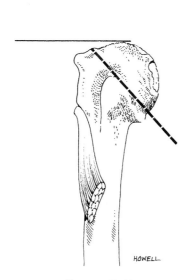

FIGURE 5-10

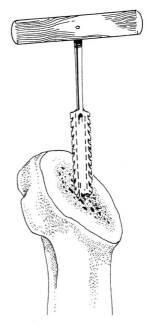

FIGURE 5-11

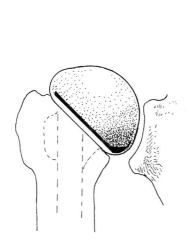

FIGURE 5-12

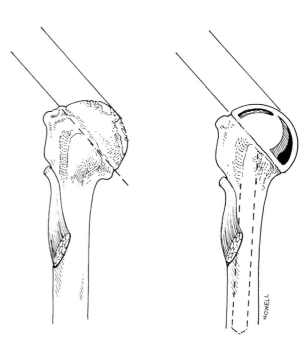

FIGURE 5-13

Next, attention is directed toward the glenoid. The key to glenoid exposure is retraction, which is aided by positioning the patient on the operating table with the glenohumeral joint extending just beyond the lateral border. It may be determined at this point that the glenoid is minimally involved, allowing use of a hemiarthroplasty. A posterior glenoid retractor is positioned to retract the osteotomized proximal humerus. Subcutaneous tissues are released at the anterior glenoid neck so that a dinner fork retractor may be placed to retract the medial structures (Fig. 5-14). This usually allows adequate visualization of the glenoid. Any soft tissue that obstructs the view, including labrum around the periphery of the glenoid, is removed. A finger should be inserted along the anterior glenoid neck to determine the location and direction of the neck and whether any osteophytes are present, which could confuse interpretation of the bony architecture. Guides are available to center the glenoid, create a longitudinal trough, or both (Fig. 5-14). With the usual Keel system, a longitudinal notch is prepared in the middle of the glenoid, being careful not to penetrate the anterior or posterior walls. The trough should enter the glenoid at right angles (Fig. 5-15). Fig. 5-16 shows an asymmetrical penetration of the glenoid wall. The trough is then deepened to receive the keel of the prosthesis, while ensuring that the anterior or posterior glenoid neck is not penetrated. The wall of the glenoid face is fashioned to roughly parallel the back wall of the glenoid component for a congruent fit. Lock key holes can be drilled into the glenoid face. Fig. 5-17 shows the sequence in glenoid preparation.

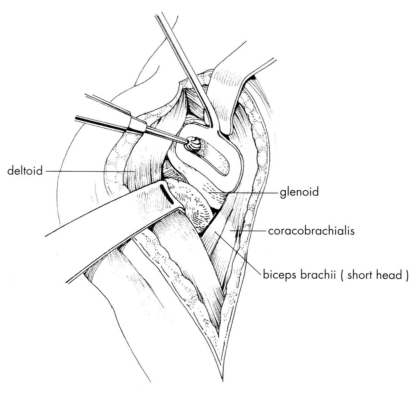

deltoid

glenoid

coracobrachialis

biceps brachii (short head)

FIGURE 5-14

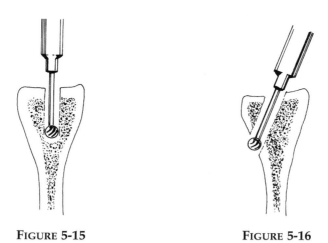

FIGURE 5-15   **FIGURE 5-16**

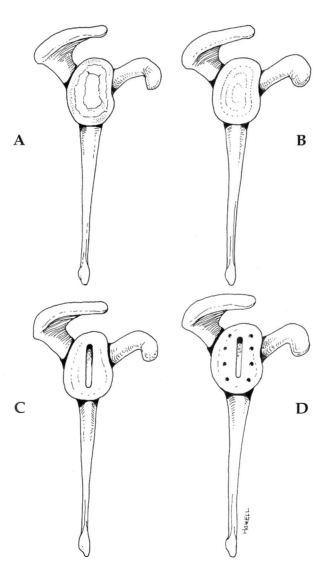

A   B

C   D

FIGURE 5-17

Once the glenoid fits securely without rocking, thrombin-soaked Gelfoam can be inserted to minimize bleeding and create an appropriate bed for cementing the glenoid component. Cement can be placed in the trough, on the back of the glenoid, or both. The glenoid is inserted and held with finger pressure. Cement should be in a doughy state before being inserted so that it will not run into the wound. Cement can be removed from the edges before it hardens. Hardened cement that is going to interfere with articulation on the edges of the glenoid can be carefully removed with a ¼-inch osteotome with sharp, clean, gentle blows. In doing this, one should try not to disengage or dislodge cement from between the posterior aspect of the glenoid prosthesis and the anterior aspect of the prepared glenoid. A finger should be passed around the cavity to ensure there are no loose pieces of cement.

Finally, the security of glenoid fixation may be tested with a Kocher clamp. The appropriate humeral stem can then be inserted into the medullary canal. If a press fit cannot be obtained, cementing is required. Before cement placement, a cement plug should be placed distally to contain the cement and aid in pressurization of the cement. The cement should be inserted with a cement gun while the cement is still fluid. During impaction of the prosthesis, care must be taken to avoid fracture of the humeral shaft, particularly in osteoporotic bone. Humeral head size is next determined. A trial reduction can be performed to select the appropriate humeral head size.

Following reduction of the components, the position, size, and version are assessed. There should be a congruent fit with the humeral head sitting opposite the glenoid face. Gentle distal longitudinal traction on the upper arm should allow one finger breadth between the acromion and the humeral head. Posterior translation, perhaps the width of the glenoid, should be possible as well as a small amount of anterior translation. Elevation and rotation should be smooth. It should be possible to close the subscapularis and capsule but still allow the desired external rotation. This assessment must be performed before final placement of the humeral component and selection of head size. Changes and adjustments can then be made. For example, if closure of the cuff is too tight, either a smaller head may be considered or more bone may be resected from the shaft.

Glenoid Preparation

Glenoid bone grafting and other considerations. If the glenoid is deficient anteriorly (Fig. 5-18), several options are available. The surgeon may build up the deficient glenoid with cement (Fig. 5-19), resect the prominent glenoid (Fig. 5-20), or less desirably, cut asymmetrically inside the glenoid and attempt to compensate by increasing the retraction (Fig. 5-21). Unfortunately, this option may lead to instability problems. A significant defect may rarely be treated with bone grafting if bone can be taken from the head, fashioned to fit in the defect, and screwed in place under a plate with one or two screws (Fig. 5-22).

Closure. The subscapularis and the rotator interval above are secured side-to-side with interrupted sutures (see Fig. 2-22). The deltopectoral interval is allowed to fall together (see Fig. 2-14). The pectoralis raphe and deltoid insertion, if incised, may be sutured. Subcutaneous tissue and skin are closed in the surgeon's preferred method over a drain.

Rotator cuff repair with shoulder arthroplasty. Occasionally, a rotator cuff defect is present and requires repair with arthroplasty. Before insertion of the humeral component, the rotator cuff is mobilized as described in Chapter 4.

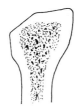

FIGURE 5-18

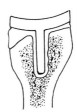

FIGURE 5-19

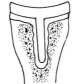

FIGURE 5-20

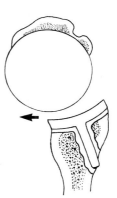

FIGURE 5-21

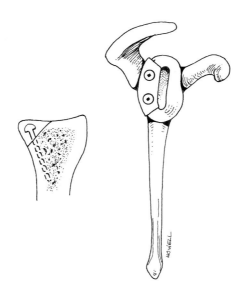

FIGURE 5-22

Once adequate mobilization is achieved, the humeral component and the head are inserted, and drill holes are placed at the level of the greater tuberosity to secure the repaired cuff defect, which may be positioned before humeral component insertion (Fig. 5-23).

POSTOPERATIVE CARE (SEE CHAPTER 11)

It is helpful to use an interscalene block and to start early motion. A passive motion machine may be used. Motion progresses from passive to active and rapidly through the phases as pain and motion allow. Phase I, or the assisted or passive program, can be carried on during the initial weeks, followed by Phase II, the active program, as soon as a reasonable good range of motion has been obtained and pain is minimal. Sometimes, the patient may return to the supine position, especially with large reconstruction, to begin active motion (Phase II). Resisted exercises are started between 4 and 8 weeks, as active motion and pain permit.

In the presence of a cuff defect, active motion is not allowed until healing has occurred, which takes approximately 6 to 8 weeks, depending on the size of the tear and the security of the repair.

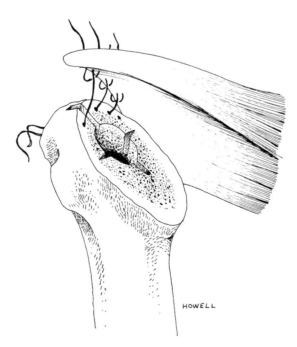

FIGURE 5-23

SPECIAL CONSIDERATIONS
Cuff Tear Arthropathy

In the presence of a cuff tear arthropathy, a large humeral head component may be inserted and the rotator cuff is not repaired. This allows articulation of the humeral component with the glenoid and the undersurface of the acromion. Acromioplasty is usually unnecessary and may be contraindicated. Pain relief is surprisingly successful in these patients. The functional return is often compromised because of the cuff deficiency.

Tuberosity Malunion

Patients with tuberosity malunion rarely require osteotomy and mobilization of the tuberosity to allow repositioning for a better functional result. In general, it is prudent not to osteotomize tuberosities unless absolutely necessary, but rather to accept malposition and insert the humeral head by working around the tuberosity malunion.

Locked Dislocations

It is important, in locked dislocations, to change the version to accommodate the postoperative tendency to subluxation. With a locked posterior dislocation, one should consider less retroversion than the normal 35° or 40°. The longer the dislocation has been present, the less retroversion that is necessary. For example, one may place the humeral component in neutral version in a patient with a locked dislocation of 1 year's duration. A similar principle applies to an anterior dislocation by increasing the retroversion of the humeral component.

Instability Patterns

Total shoulder arthroplasty can be performed in the presence of instability. The Neer system, for example, is more constrained than a normal glenohumeral joint and, therefore, can restore stability. Where indicated, additional soft tissue balancing may be added to increase stability. Humeral version adjustments can help compensate for instability tendencies.

Arthrodesis
GENERAL CONSIDERATIONS
Indications

Occasionally, neurological disorders of the shoulder, such as brachial plexus lesions and other palsies, may still be an indication for glenohumeral arthrodesis. A more common indication is the very painful multioperated shoulder when no other alternatives are available, for example, following failed cuff or instability surgery.

Contraindications

A contraindication may be the existence of nonfunctioning scapular muscles. The scapulothoracic articulation is the only motor for the shoulder girdle in the presence of a glenohumeral arthrodesis.

Expectations

The expectations following arthrodesis are limited. The functional outcome is poor, with ability to perform daily living activities often compromised. Work can usually be performed only at the waist level. Lifting at waist level is also possible. Unfortunately, some pain is frequently present after an arthrodesis, especially if there is any element of scapular winging causing scapulothoracic pain. Cosmetically, it is somewhat disfiguring. It is, therefore, a "last resort" operation when nothing else is available and pain is intolerable. We often precede arthrodesis with the use of a shoulder spica for 1 to 2 weeks to get a measure of pain relief, which may correlate with the pain relief that would be obtained with fusion.

SURGICAL TECHNIQUE
Positioning

The approach for arthrodesis can be anterior or posterior and, therefore, positioning can be in the "beach chair" (see Fig. 2-1) or the prone position (see Fig. 2-3). Our preference is the lateral decubitus position (see Fig. 2-4). This position allows a posterior approach, which provides an appreciation of the glenoid neck orientation for screw placement.

Approach

The posterior approach is the easiest and most technically feasible approach. The incision extends along the spine of the scapula over the lateral border of the acromion and distally along the anterolateral aspect of the humeral shaft (Fig. 5-24).

Procedure

The deltoid muscle is dissected from most of the acromion to allow adequate exposure of the underlying rotator cuff (Fig. 5-25). It may be prudent to not violate neurological structures in the unlikely event that subsequent neurological function, such as axillary nerve function, is required. Arthrodeses have been taken down and total shoulders inserted; however, that would be very rarely indicated. The rotator cuff is excised in its entirety as it overlies the humeral head to allow denuding of the cartilaginous surfaces for subsequent fusion of humeral head to glenoid and humeral head to the undersurface of the acromion. The undersurface of the acromion is denuded of periosteum down to bleeding bone with the use of a power burr (Fig. 5-26).

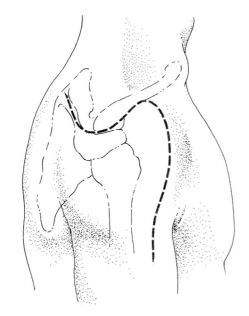

FIGURE 5-24

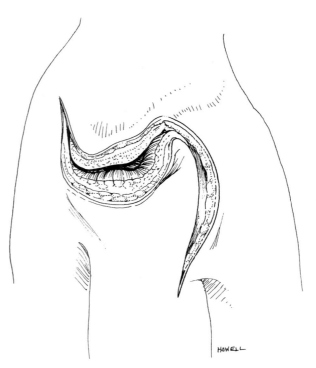

FIGURE 5-25

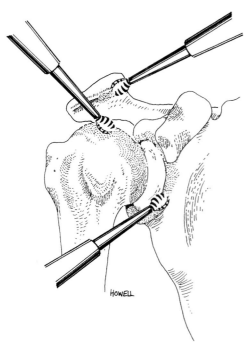

FIGURE 5-26

Similarly, the articular surface may be removed from the humeral head and the glenoid with a power burr, or osteotomy cuts can be planned to fit the humeral head to the glenoid. We have found that denuding the articular surface of the humeral head glenoid in its own configuration allows the best fit. It is important to remember the position of arthrodesis in preparing osteotomy cuts and performing the burring.

During the procedure, the shoulder can be positioned in approximately 10° to 20° of forward flexion, 20° to 40° of abduction, and approximately 35 to 40° of internal rotation (Fig. 5-27), which is achieved by allowing the hand to reach the mouth while the other positions are maintained. The ideal position is seldom exactly achieved, and it is through trial and error that one is eventually satisfied with the position.

There are several methods of fixation for the arthrodesis. The simplest method uses the large cancellous screws from the tuberosity into the humeral head into the glenoid. With osteotomy of the spine of the scapula, the posterior acromion can be tilted inferiorly, and screws can be inserted from the acromion into the humeral head. The addition of a large 3.5 reconstruction plate allows more security, requiring less postoperative immobilization time. The plate adds operative time and, because of its prominence, may have to be removed in patients who have wasted musculature. The plate may be necessary in patients who cannot tolerate prolonged immobilization.

Following contouring of the bony surfaces, the humeral head is secured to the glenoid by three pins for large fragment cannulated drill bits. The pins should be placed in as divergent a manner as possible (Fig. 5-28). The surgeon can reposition the pins if the position is unsatisfactory. The pins are then overdrilled and tapped, and large fragment cancellous screws with washers are inserted (Fig. 5-29). By placing fingers along the anterior and posterior glenoid neck, one can get an appreciation for the appropriate direction of the cancellous screws. The correct direction will avoid violating the glenoid neck margins and will keep the screws within the glenoid neck (Fig. 5-30).

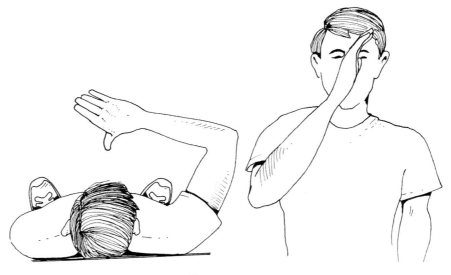

FIGURE 5-27

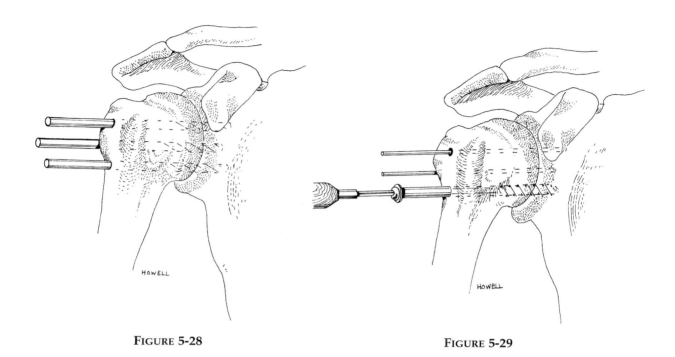

FIGURE 5-28   **FIGURE 5-29**

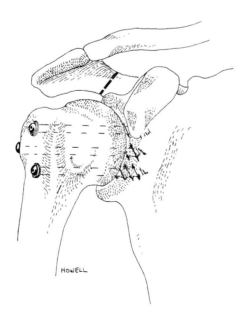

FIGURE 5-30

Positioning of the humeral head as superiorly as possible will lessen the distance the spine must be pushed inferiorly with an osteotomy. However, superior placement of the humeral head also decreases the contact area between the head and the glenoid, which is very important. Therefore, it is usually necessary at this point to osteotomize the spine of the scapula and bend the posterior acromion down to the humeral head, trying to fit it appropriately with as much bone contact as possible (Figs. 5-30 and 5-31). Two large fragment cancellous screws are inserted from the acromion into the humeral head (Fig. 5-32). If a reconstruction plate is applied, it is contoured along the spine of the scapula over the acromion and the humeral head and down the proximal shaft of the humerus with appropriate screw fixation (Fig. 5-33). A 3.5 reconstruction plate can be used in smaller patients and a 4.5 plate for larger patients.

Closure

The deltoid is reapproximated to its origin through drill holes, if necessary, and subcutaneous tissue and skin are closed in the preferred method of the surgeon. A drain is normally used.

POSTOPERATIVE CARE (SEE CHAPTER 11)

The postoperative care for an arthrodesis generally involves immobilization. If a reconstruction plate is used along with the cancellous screws in the glenoid, sometimes immobilization time can be lessened. It is still advisable, even in this circumstance, to immobilize the shoulder for 6 weeks. If cancellous screws alone are used, the immobilization period should approach 12 weeks. Upon removal of immobilization, a sling should be applied and gentle pendulum exercises performed. As the fusion becomes secure, motion can be initiated in the shoulder girdle, which should focus on the scapulothoracic articulation. Strengthening of the scapular muscles can be instituted once the fusion becomes secure.

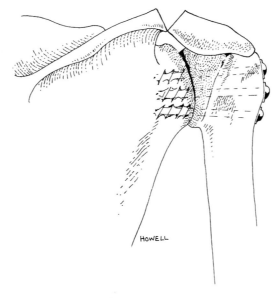

FIGURE 5-31

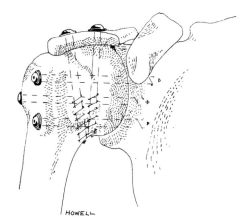

FIGURE 5-32

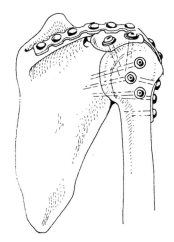

FIGURE 5-33

Neurological Disorders and Muscle Transfers

6

Introduction

It is unusual to have to approach a neurological lesion or perform a muscle transfer about the shoulder. The common neurological lesions seen about the shoulder that might require surgery relate to the axillary nerve, suprascapular nerve, brachial plexus, and long thoracic nerve. These lesions may occasionally lead to the need for some form of nerve surgery, muscle transfers, or scapular stabilizing procedures. A pectoralis rupture might also require repair, reconstruction, or both.

Suprascapular Nerve Decompression

GENERAL CONSIDERATIONS

A suprascapular nerve lesion can begin traumatically or spontaneously as a result of compression as it goes through the suprascapular notch or around the spinoglenoid notch. In patients with a painful shoulder with obvious involvement of both the infraspinatus and the supraspinatus, the pathology is at the suprascapular notch. If the infraspinatus alone is involved, pathology occurs more laterally as the nerve winds around the spinoglenoid notch, often a result of a spinoglenoid notch cyst. There may be associated weakness of external rotation and, sometimes, abduction of the shoulder. Electromyogram (EMG) and nerve conduction studies are necessary to document the compression. Treatment is usually conservative because spontaneous recovery usually occurs. Occasionally, decompression is indicated for pain relief and functional improvement when there is no evidence of recovery. The timing of such surgery is important, but unclear, although perhaps should be considered with the appropriate symptoms and no improvement, either clinically or electromyographically, for 3 months.

Sometimes, release of the suprascapular notch alone is adequate if compression is at that level. Sometimes, the spinoglenoid notch also requires attention if, for example, there is a spinoglenoid notch cyst. Sometimes, only that cyst requires attention.

If the pathology is isolated to the suprascapular notch, two options of surgical approach are available. If the pathology is a spinoglenoid notch cyst with some nerve compression, a specific approach is necessary. Alternatively, if pathology seems to be at both levels, the suprascapular notch and the spinoglenoid notch, a larger exposure is required to deal with both areas.

Indications

The indication for release of the suprascapular notch is a painful and/or functionally disabling weak shoulder with EMG documentation of suprascapular nerve entrapment and failure to improve with time. The question of timing is controversial, somewhat symptomatic, and depends on an EMG. Most such entrapments resolve with nonoperative treatment.

Expectations

The expectations, as with many neurological releases, are guarded, depending on symptoms, duration, and degree. The less involved and earlier the surgery, the more favorable the outcome. The longer the duration of symptoms, particularly in the presence of significant weakness, the more guarded the outcome, particularly as it relates to restoration of strength.

SURGICAL TECHNIQUE
Positioning

The patient may be placed in the lateral position (see Fig. 2-3) so that both the superior aspect of the supraspinatus fossa and the posterior aspect of the spinoglenoid notch can be approached. For an isolated approach to the suprascapular notch, the patient can be placed in the "beach chair" (see Fig. 2-1) or semi-sitting (see Fig. 2-2) position, with appropriate draping to allow an approach to the supraspinatus fossa.

Approach with Vertical Incision to Suprascapular Notch

In the supine position, the vertical incision is approximately 2.5 cm long, extending from the clavicle anteriorly to the spine of the scapula posteriorly (Fig. 6-1, a). It is two finger breadths medial to the apex of the junction of the clavicle and the spine, that is, the supraspinous arthroscopy portal. A further landmark for this incision is that its anterior extent is at the level of the coracoid. A transverse incision is also an option (Fig. 6-1, b) (described in the next section).

Procedure

The trapezius muscle overlying the supraspinatus fossa is spread in the direction of its fibers, revealing the underlying supraspinatus muscle fibers. The supraspinatus muscle fibers are spread, and with finger dissection, the area of the suprascapular notch is palpated (Fig. 6-2). With caution and patience, the notch can be identified and the suprascapular ligament can be released. Identification of the nerve with this limited exposure is difficult.

Closure

The supraspinatus muscle fibers and trapezius muscle fibers fall together. The subcutaneous tissue and skin are closed in the manner the surgeon prefers. Use of a drain is unnecessary.

POSTOPERATIVE CARE (SEE CHAPTER 11)

The patient may progress rapidly from Phase I to Phase II to Phase III of the rehabilitation program. Eventual emphasis should be on concentric and eccentric strengthening of the rotators, particularly the infraspinatus.

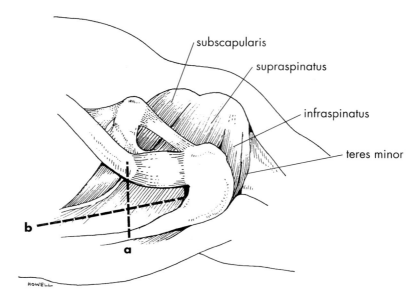

FIGURE 6-1

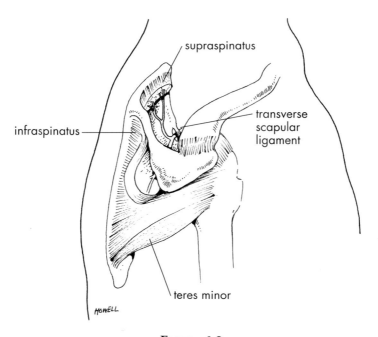

FIGURE 6-2

Approach with Transverse Incision to Suprascapular Notch Position

The position for the transverse incision may be either supine (especially semi-sitting) (see Fig 2-2) or lateral. The lateral position allows more extensive exposure (see Fig. 2-4) if the spinoglenoid notch must be approached. The incision is approximately 4 cm long in a transverse direction, extending along the spine of the scapula, beginning laterally at the apex of the clavicle and scapular spine (Fig. 6-1, *b*), that is, the Neveiser arthroscopy portal (see Fig. 10-6).

Procedure

The trapezius is reflected off the spine. The underlying supraspinatus is identified, and dissection is directed down the spine, mobilizing the muscle anteriorly until the floor of the fossa is reached (Fig. 6-3). The supraspinatus muscle is elevated and retracted anteriorly until the nerve and notch are identified. The ligament is then released.

Closure

The supraspinatus muscle falls back into its bed. The trapezius is reapproximated over the spine. Subcutaneous tissue and skin are closed as the surgeon prefers. A drain is usually not required.

POSTOPERATIVE CARE (SEE CHAPTER 11)

The patient may progress rapidly from Phase I to Phase II to Phase III of the rehabilitation program. Eventual emphasis should be on concentric and eccentric strengthening of the rotators, particularly the infraspinatus.

Spinoglenoid Notch Cyst Approach

A spinoglenoid notch cyst may require surgical approach. Initially, a needle may be used to decompress the cyst. Failing that, if there is a posterior superior labral lesion, unroofing of that lesion arthroscopically may decompress the cyst since they frequently communicate. Failing that, the following surgical approach to excise the cyst may be required.

Positioning

The lateral decubitus position is probably the most advantageous, allowing an extensive approach, particularly posteriorly to the level of the spinoglenoid notch cyst (see Fig. 2-4).

Incision Approach

The incision is transverse, approximately 4 cm long, just inferior to the spine of the scapula curving downward laterally toward the axilla. The supraspinatus muscle can be reflected anteriorly, to identify the suprascapular nerve in the floor of the supraspinatus fossa (Fig. 6-3). The supraspinatus fossa can be followed to the spinoglenoid notch, at which time the cyst may be identified (Fig. 6-4). From this level, the cyst can be decompressed and excised. If one wishes only to go posteriorly to the spinoglenoid notch, a vertical incision (Fig. 6-1, *a*) extending more posteriorly could be used. If it is an enlarged cyst extending around the corner of the spinoglenoid notch, the deltoid will require reflection off the spine of the scapula distally to identify the underlying infraspinatus muscle (Fig. 6-4). With finger palpation around the corner of the cyst, the infraspinatus muscle can be spread apart and the cyst identified and excised distally if it extends around the notch.

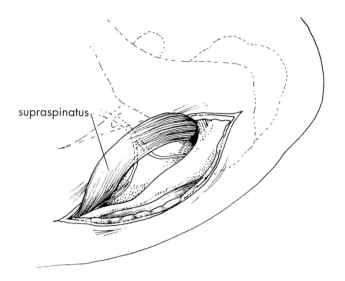

supraspinatus

FIGURE 6-3

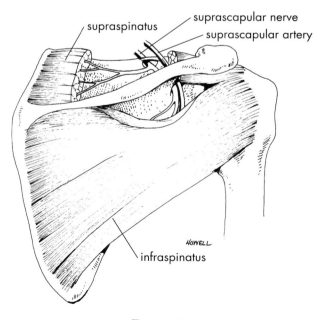

supraspinatus   suprascapular nerve

suprascapular artery

infraspinatus

FIGURE 6-4

Closure

The deltoid must be resutured to the spine of the glenoid through drill holes, if necessary. The remainder of the musculature simply falls together, while the subcutaneous tissue and skin are closed in the surgeon's preferred manner. Use of a drain is unnecessary.

POSTOPERATIVE CARE (SEE CHAPTER 11)

The patient may progress rapidly from Phase I to Phase II to Phase III of the rehabilitation program. Eventual emphasis should be on concentric and eccentric strengthening of the rotators, particularly the infraspinatus.

The postoperative course consists of early range of motion exercises, progressing rapidly through the phases with emphasis on external rotation strengthening, both concentric and eccentric.

SCAPULAR WINGING

Scapular winging can be caused by a long thoracic nerve palsy knocking out the serratus anterior muscle or an accessory nerve palsy knocking out the trapezius muscle. It can also be biomechanically related to non-neurological shoulder pathology. The procedures for scapular winging are many. Perhaps the most common is a pectoralis major transfer. A pectoralis minor transfer and various forms of fascial slings are also used. Scapulothoracic arthrodesis may be an option in select cases of scapular winging, particularly those associated with fascial-scapulohumeral dystrophy. Trapezius palsy can cause scapular winging, which often follows biopsy of a lymph node in the supraclavicular fossa. The procedure for correction of this palsy is the Whitman procedure, which consists of a transfer of the rhomboids and levator scapulae medially, securing them onto the scapula. Because of the "scapular lag" with winging, there may be secondary impingement. Most cases of scapular winging, especially with long thoracic involvement, resolve with time.

Pectoralis Major Transfer for Scapular Winging
GENERAL CONSIDERATIONS
Indications

The indication for pectoralis major transfer with fascial or synthetic extension is symptomatic scapular winging for a prolonged period (1 year) usually a result of serratus anterior palsy related to a long thoracic nerve deficiency.

Expectations

The expectations regarding this procedure would be to effectively diminish the scapular winging and to return near normal function to the shoulder, although with some degree of mild weakness. Pain, if present, is often relieved. The repair occasionally stretches out with time, allowing for some recurrence of winging, but function often remains intact. Laboring workers often do not return to such work. Improvement, therefore, is seldom to normal.

SURGICAL TECHNIQUE
Position

The patient is best placed in the lateral decubitus position (see Fig. 2-4). The arm should be draped free. The left thigh is draped free to take a fascial graft. We have occasionally used synthetic materials for the fascial extension.

Approach

The incision extends from distally, beginning at the inferior angle of the scapula, running along the lateral border of the scapular into the axilla to the anterior pectoral fold, and half way up the deltopectoral interval (Fig. 6-5).

Procedure

The deltopectoral interval is identified (see Fig. 2-14), and the tendinous sternal portion of the head of the pectoralis major is dissected from its origin adjacent and inferior to the lesser tuberosity. A fascial graft is taken from the thigh, approximately 1 in. in diameter and approximately 8 to 10 in. long. The length of fascia graft required is often less than expected. It is tubed and sewn onto itself. After dissecting the tendinous portion of the pectoralis off the bone, the fascial strip is sutured onto the distal tendon (Fig. 6-6). The fascial strip is passed directly adjacent to the rib cage under the skin. It exits posteriorly at the lower border of the scapula (Fig. 6-7). The serratus is identified on the lateral inferior border of the scapula. It is dissected free to identify the inferior pole of the scapula, and a drill hole is made in the mid-portion inferiorly in the scapula, approximately 1 in. from its tip. The fascial strip is passed through the drill holes from deep to superficial and sutured back onto itself, holding the scapula in a quite secure tenodesis fashion (Fig. 6-8). It should be snug enough to pull the inferior pole slightly laterally.

Closure

The wounds are closed in the usual fashion. The use of a drain is optional, but usually unnecessary.

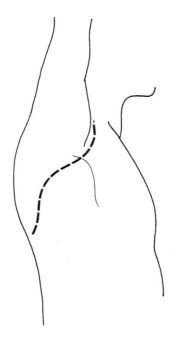

FIGURE 6-5

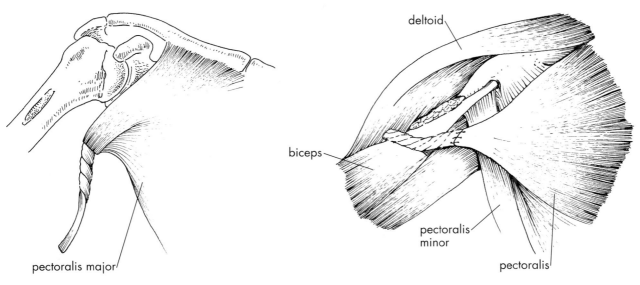

pectoralis major

FIGURE 6-6

deltoid

biceps

pectoralis
minor

pectoralis

FIGURE 6-7

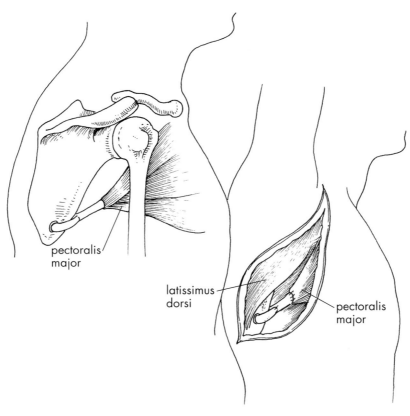

pectoralis
major

latissimus
dorsi

pectoralis
major

FIGURE 6-8

POSTOPERATIVE CARE (SEE CHAPTER 11)

Postoperative care consists of temporary immobilization in a sling for 3 to 4 weeks, followed by gentle range of motion exercises. Initially assisted, motion becomes active in a couple of weeks, followed by resisted exercises (particularly serratus-type strengthening with seated rows, shrugs, push-ups) and rotational exercises for the shoulder.

Levator and Rhomboid Transfer for Scapular Winging Caused by Trapezius Palsy

GENERAL CONSIDERATIONS

Indications

The indications for this transfer relate to scapular winging caused by trapezius knock-out, which can be functionally disabling and sometimes painful. Pain can be a result of both the winging and, sometimes, of an associated impingement tendinitis.

Expectations

The expectations following this surgery are restoration of more normal scapular mechanics and lessening of the discomfort. The operation is rarely indicated and rarely performed.

SURGICAL TECHNIQUE

Positioning

The patient is placed either prone or, more advantageously, in the lateral decubitus position (see Fig. 2-4). The arm is draped free.

Procedure

A longitudinal incision is made along the medial border of the scapula from just proximal to the inferior tip to approximately 1 in. above the spine (Fig. 6-9).

The major and minor rhomboid muscles and their insertion into the medial border of the scapula are identified. Superiorly, the trapezius is dissected from the spine of the scapula, and the underlying levator scapulae are identified (Fig. 6-10). Care must be taken regarding the accessory nerve as it courses adjacent to the levator scapulae, but it is likely already deficient as a result of the pathology.

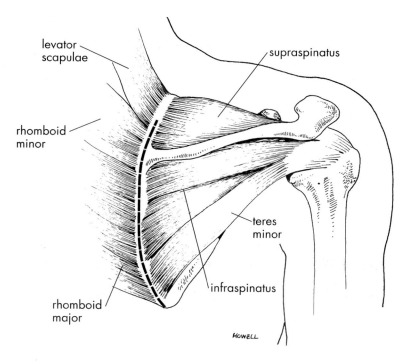

FIGURE 6-9

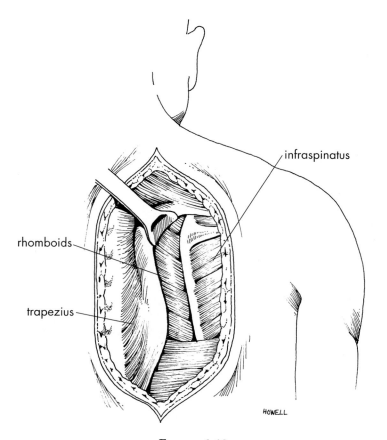

FIGURE 6-10

Both the major and the minor rhomboids are removed from the medial border of the scapula, taking a thin piece of bone and periosteum with their insertions (Fig. 6-11). Similarly, the levator scapulae is removed from the spine of the scapula and the upper medial border with a sliver of bone and periosteum, which is very important for fixation. The infraspinatus muscle is elevated off the scapula, and the rhomboids are transferred medially a distance of 3 to 4 cm (Fig. 6-12). The levator scapulae is similarly transferred medially and then sutured, mattress fashion, through drill holes in bone with some slight roughening of the bone of the scapula to create a better bed for healing (Fig. 6-12).

Closure

The infraspinatus is closed over the repair. Subcutaneous tissue and skin are closed as the surgeon prefers. The use of a drain is optional.

POSTOPERATIVE CARE (SEE CHAPTER 11)

The patient is immobilized with the arm in slight forward elevation and abduction on a pillow or in a brace for 6 weeks. Gentle passive exercises may be started above the level of the brace or pillow. When the brace is removed, Phase II active exercises are followed by resisted exercises within a few weeks.

Scapulothoracic Arthrodesis
GENERAL CONSIDERATIONS
Indications

Scapulothoracic arthrodesis is rarely indicated. It may be used in patients who have fascioscapulohumeral dystrophy or may occasionally be attempted in patients who have symptomatic scapular winging, particularly global. Pain relief is the usual indication, although functional improvement may be seen in patients with fascioscapulohumeral dystrophy.

Expectations

The expectation regarding arthrodesis is a surprisingly functional range of motion of the shoulder with reasonable functional capacity for daily living activities and even light work.

SURGICAL TECHNIQUE
Positioning

The patient is placed in a prone position. The scapula is draped beyond its medial border over to the midline, and the arm is draped free.

Approach

An incision is made along the medial border of the scapula from superior to the spine down to the inferior angle (see Fig. 6-9). The trapezius is retracted medially (see Fig. 6-10) The rhomboid muscles are incised subperiosteally and off the edge of the scapula to allow subsequent reattachment.

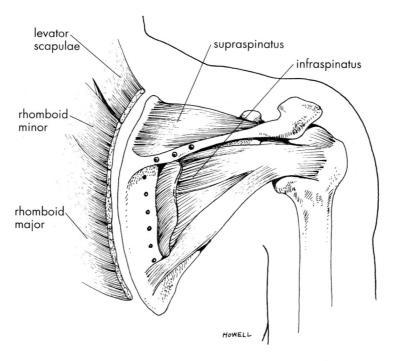

FIGURE 6-11

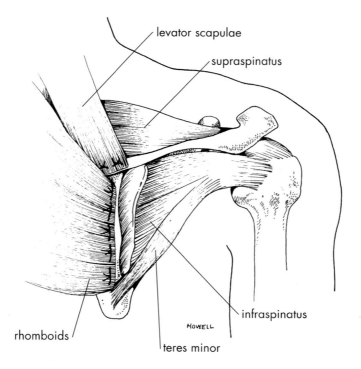

FIGURE 6-12

Procedure

Once the rhomboid muscles are elevated, the scapula can be lifted away from the rib cage. The soft tissue of the serratus and subscapularis is resected off the under-surface aspect of the scapula, down to denuded bone, which is slightly roughened with a burr. The ribs are carefully identified following resection of muscle, and the periosteum is incised in a longitudinal direction. The periosteum is carefully stripped off of ribs four, five, and six, posteriorly. The ribs are denuded with a burr down to bleeding bone (Fig. 6-13) over as wide an area as possible. This takes into account the final position of the scapula, which will lie in 20° to 25° of external rotation to maximize the subsequent range of elevation and external rotation. After using rib and periosteal dissectors, a 19-gauge wire is carefully passed around each of the exposed ribs (Fig. 6-14). Drill holes are made in the scapula, which is positioned in approximately 20° to 25° of external rotation, lining up the drill holes with their corresponding wires (Fig. 6-15). Cancellous bone is taken from the posterior iliac crest. A semitubular type of plate is then flattened to go over the scapula, lining it up appropriately with the drill holes. The plate allows adequate stress distribution. The bone graft is inserted under the scapula (Fig. 6-16). The drill holes receive the wire, and the plate and the scapula are secured to the ribs (Fig. 6-17) in some external rotation. The rhomboids are reattached.

Closure

The subcutaneous tissue and skin are closed in the usual fashion. It would be appropriate to insert a drain. A postoperative x-ray to rule out pneumothorax is advisable.

POSTOPERATIVE CARE (SEE CHAPTER 11)

A simple sling is applied postoperatively. In a few days, a spica is applied to immobilize the upper extremity for 12 weeks. This is followed by gentle range of motion exercises, progressing through the phases fairly rapidly from passive to active to resisted.

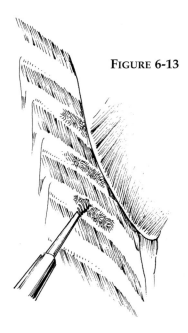

FIGURE 6-13

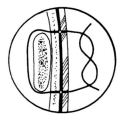

FIGURE 6-14

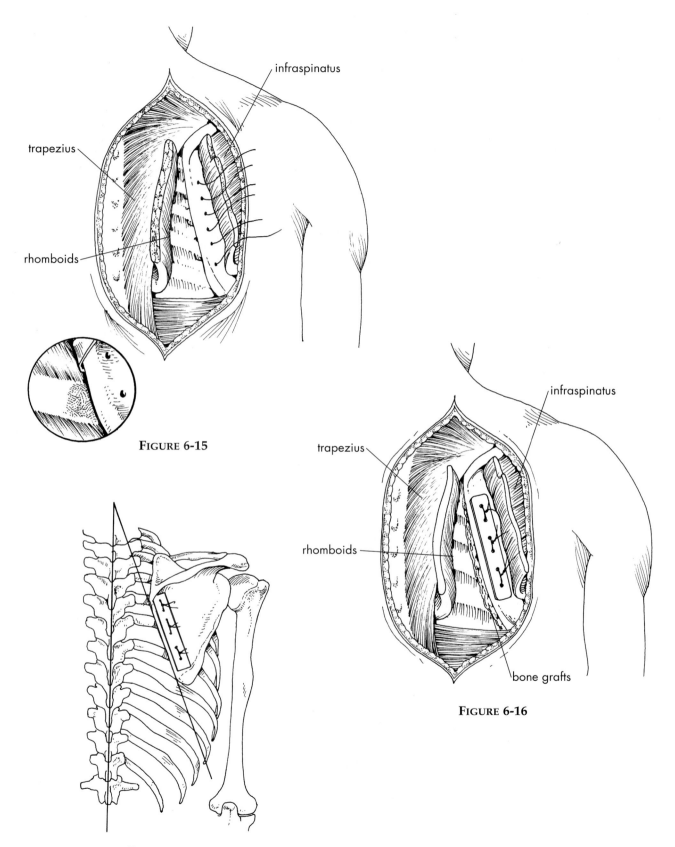

infraspinatus

trapezius

rhomboids

FIGURE 6-15

infraspinatus

trapezius

rhomboids

bone grafts

FIGURE 6-16

FIGURE 6-17

Pectoralis Muscle Repair
GENERAL CONSIDERATIONS

The pectoralis muscle tendon unit can rupture, almost always from the humeral insertion, during an eccentric overload usually on the externally rotated and abducted and extended arm.

Indications

The indications for repair are a symptomatic deformity for an acute or sometimes late rupture. It may be repaired as late as 18 months following the injury. Certain athletes such as gymnasts have a particular functional disability related to a pectoralis rupture if it is not repaired early to restore normal function.

Expectations

The expectations following such a procedure are restoration of near normal contour, albeit with some slight deformity, and near normal function and strength.

SURGICAL TECHNIQUE
Positioning

The patient is placed in the "beach chair" (see Fig. 2-1) or semi-sitting position (see Fig. 2-2). An inflatable cuff may be placed under the ipsilateral shoulder. The right arm is draped free.

Approach

The skin incision is a deltopectoral approach (see Fig. 2-9), slightly distal to the usual approach. The interval is easily identified (see Fig. 2-14), and sometimes the medial wall is deficient because of the absent, ruptured, and medially retracted pectoralis.

Procedure

Both ends can be ruptured, but it is often only the underlying deep head. If approached early, the pathology is usually evident (Fig. 6-18). If approached late, dissection may be required to excise scar tissue and identify the retracted and scarred tendon. The tendon is mobilized after it is dissected free. Adjacent to the lesser tuberosity and biceps, the humeral shaft is exposed and roughened. Drill holes are made and the tendon sutured to the drill holes through four or five secure sutures (Fig. 6-19). An anchoring system could be used for such a repair.

Closure

The subcutaneous tissue and skin are closed as the surgeon prefers. Use of a drain is optional but seldom necessary.

POSTOPERATIVE CARE (SEE CHAPTER 11)

The patient is immobilized in a simple sling with the forearm across the chest for 4 weeks. During that time, gentle shoulder elevation, internal rotation, and pendulum exercises may be used. At 4 weeks, more aggressive elevation and internal rotation along with external rotation to neutral may be undertaken. At 6 weeks, active exercises are started, followed shortly thereafter by gentle internal rotation concentric and eccentric strengthening. During this time, external rotation is gradually stretched to return to normal by 12 weeks, at which time aggressive concentric and particularly eccentric strengthening of the pectoralis is emphasized.

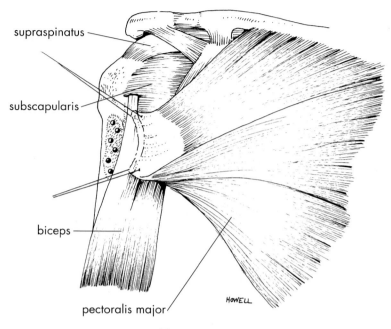

supraspinatus

subscapularis

biceps

pectoralis major

HOWELL

FIGURE 6-18

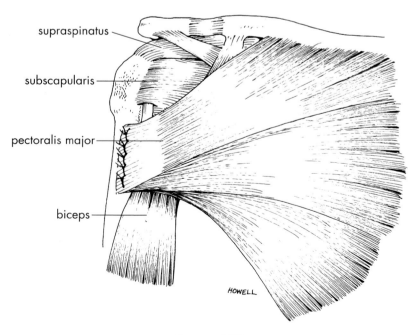

supraspinatus

subscapularis

pectoralis major

biceps

HOWELL

FIGURE 6-19

Fractures

7

Introduction

The majority of proximal humeral fractures (85%) are nondisplaced, requiring temporary immobilization for 2 to 3 weeks followed by a carefully monitored rehabilitation program. The remaining 15% of proximal humeral fractures are displaced, ranging from isolated displaced greater tuberosity fractures to complex fracture dislocations requiring hemiarthroplasty.

Although various classifications exist, for purposes of uniformity and standardization, most orthopaedic surgeons in North America apply Neer's classification system. This system has some shortcomings in that not all variations of fracture patterns are addressed. This system is based on a definition of displacement being more than 1 cm, greater than 45° of angulation, or both. Four segments are involved in this fracture classification system: the head, the greater tuberosity, the lesser tuberosity, and the shaft. In addition, there may be an associated dislocation. For a fracture to be more than a one-part fracture, the previously mentioned displacement must be present, either of a separate piece (that is, the shaft) or of a group of smaller pieces (that is, fragmented greater tuberosity). Two-part fractures will typically be either a displaced surgical neck fracture or a displaced greater tuberosity fracture. Rarely, anatomical neck fractures, lesser tuberosity fractures, or both will occur. Three-part fractures consist of a displaced surgical neck fracture and a rotated, displaced head fragment, usually with attached lesser tuberosity and displaced greater tuberosity. Occasionally, the lesser tuberosity will be avulsed with the greater tuberosity still intact on the head fragment. Four-part fractures consist of either a displaced surgical neck or an anatomical neck fracture with a displaced head fragment and displaced greater and lesser tuberosity fractures.

The importance of this classification rests not only in the surgeon's ability to categorize fracture types but, more importantly, to determine appropriate treatment. To appropriately classify these fractures, adequate radiographic studies are essential. A standard trauma series consisting of a true AP view, a scapular lateral view, and an axillary view will allow such classification. Although the AP and scapular lateral views are readily obtained, the axillary view may be more challenging. Several options exist. An IV tree on wheels is brought to the side of the patient's bed and the patient is asked to grasp the IV pole with the involved arm. By means of gentle abduction moving the pole away from the bed, with the x-ray plate above the shoulder, the beam is then brought into the axilla for the axillary view. If the patient is unable to cooperate, a Velpeau axillary may be obtained. In this view, with the patient standing, he or she is asked to lean back over the x-ray table so that the involved shoulder will lie beneath the beam, which is directed from above toward the table. Although this does not give the clarity and definition of a true axillary view, it is sufficient in certain situations. True AP and axillary views are the best views to determine the fracture pattern.

This chapter will discuss the surgical treatment of two-part, three-part, and four-part fractures. In addition to these proximal humeral fractures, scapular and clavicle fractures will be discussed.

Open Reduction of Two-Part Fractures (Greater Tuberosity)
GENERAL CONSIDERATIONS

Greater tuberosity fractures typically occur in association with anterior subcoracoid dislocations. In most cases the tuberosity will reduce anatomically with the shoulder reduction. These fractures rarely remain displaced, implying an associated longitudinal cuff defect. They seldom require open reduction. Radiographical studies should be used to determine the degree of superior lateral, as well as posterior, displacement. Displacement of this fracture is attributable to its rotator cuff attachment, specifically the supraspinatus and infraspinatus, resulting in a component of superior and posterior displacement. The superior displacement is best seen on the AP view, while the posterior displacement may be demonstrated on the lateral view and optimally on the axillary view. Occasionally, a CT scan may be helpful in further defining not only the displacement but also the degree of comminution and possible involvement of the posterior portion of the glenoid articular surface.

Superiorly displaced greater tuberosity fractures that are left displaced in active, healthy patients will often result in chronic impingement and significant functional limitations. Given the displacement patterns that have been discussed previously, those individuals meeting the criteria of a two-part fracture may be readily treated by several means of internal fixation, such as cannulated screws, wire sutures, or pins.

Indications

Ideal candidates for open reduction of two-part fractures are active patients with displaced greater tuberosity fractures. Poor bone quality or questionable medical status may be relative contraindications that should be evaluated on an individual basis.

Expectations

With an anatomical repair of the cuff and tuberosity, as a rule, one should see a return to nearly full motion and function.

SURGICAL TECHNIQUE
Positioning

The patient is placed in a "beach chair" (see Fig. 2-1) or semi-sitting (see Fig. 2-2) position with the arm draped free. An inflatable pillow or a 500-cc IV bag is placed under the ipsilateral shoulder to bring it into a more advantageous position to approach. If cannulated screws are used for fixation of a tuberosity fracture, the patient must be placed on a frame suitable for fluoroscopy. Placing the body with the entire shoulder girdle off to the side of the table may be adequate.

Approach

The approach uses either a vertical or transverse incision for exposure of the lateral aspect of the proximal humerus (see Fig. 2-35). A vertical incision begins 1 cm posterior to the anterolateral corner of the acromion and 1 cm medial to the lateral margin. The incision is brought down vertically in line with the deltoid fibers for approximately 3 to 4 cm (see Fig. 2-35, *a*). A transverse incision may also be used to orient the incision with Langer's lines (see Fig. 2-35, *b*). However, we have not found this to be cosmetically necessary. With the skin incised, the deltoid fascia is readily identified (Fig. 7-1), and its fibers are split 3 to 4 cm distally from the acromion. A tag suture may be placed at the inferior extent of the deltoid split to prevent progression (Fig. 7-2). Furthermore, the surgeon is cautioned against vigorous distal dissection in the deltoid because of the proximity of the axillary nerve as it passes around the lateral aspect of the arm.

The tuberosity is usually noted to be superiorly and posteriorly displaced. To facilitate mobilization, traction sutures are placed in the two inferior corners of the greater tuberosity fragment (Fig. 7-2). If an associated rent in the cuff is present, it must be identified. In most instances, there will be a tear that begins at the rotator cuff interval, between subscapularis and supraspinatus, extending medially. This extension allows the superior and posterior translation of the greater tuberosity (Fig. 7-3). Once the tuberosity fragment is appropriately reduced, the internal fixation may be achieved through several methods. One technique is AO instrumentation using cannulated screws. This technique may be aided with image intensification in the AP and axillary views. This technique begins with placement of threaded guide wires perpendicular to the fracture and aimed in a somewhat antegrade fashion toward the inferior portion of the humeral head. This placement avoids the risk of penetration of the screws through the articular surface of the humeral head.

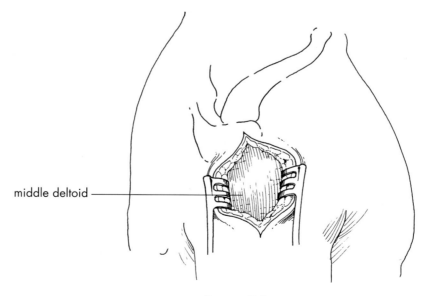

middle deltoid ———

FIGURE 7-1

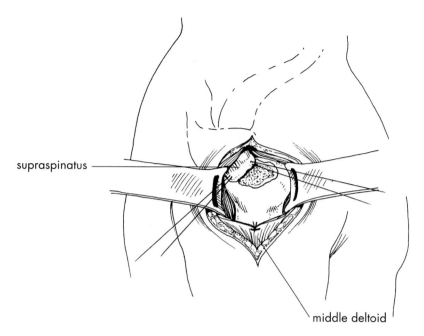

supraspinatus

middle deltoid

FIGURE 7-2

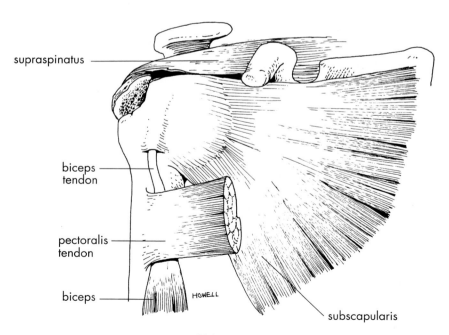

supraspinatus

biceps
tendon

pectoralis
tendon

biceps

subscapularis

FIGURE 7-3

In most cases, the direction of the guide wires will, however, be determined by the location of the fracture and obliquity of the outer cortical surface. If the guide wire is directed inferiorly toward the metaphyseal area, a second cortex may be captured. If the screws are simply placed into the humeral head, fixation relies solely on the cancellous bone of the humeral head, which may be of poor quality.

With the guide wire placed and films or fluoroscopy confirming not only reduction of the fracture but also position of the guide wires, standard AO technique is used to place two screws. These screws may be placed vertically or horizontally according to the fragment orientation (Fig. 7-4). If the quality of the bone is in question, washers should be used. Washers may be further augmented with cortical sutures about the margins of the tuberosity. Fig. 7-4 shows the anterior view of the oblique orientation of the screws to capture the second cortex in the metaphyseal portion of the humerus. If this orientation is impossible, the screws may be directed more centrally, realizing though that fixation then relies on the cancellous portion of the humeral head. The screws are not fully threaded, which allows a lag effect for compression at the fracture site. If necessary, the rotator cuff defect is repaired to complete the procedure (Fig. 7-5).

An alternate technique to screw fixation is that of tension band wiring (Fig. 7-6). It is ideally suited to this situation because the fracture occurs on the tension side of the humerus, near the insertion of the rotator cuff tendons. By predrilling the humeral shaft and bringing the AO cerclage wire or cable grip material up under the insertion of the rotator cuff and into the greater tuberosity fragment, a stable construct may be established. The tendon of the supraspinatus is captured in the repair. This technique is suitable for individuals with porotic bone or excessive comminution.

In those individuals in whom screw fixation is deemed inappropriate or fails, multiple nonabsorbable sutures around the tuberosity fragment may be adequate to initially stabilize the fracture. As shown in Fig. 7-7, this technique may require more prolonged immobilization because of a potentially tenuous repair. However, in individuals with reasonable quality cortical bone, reasonable stability may be obtained and early motion used by predrilling the suture sites, thus avoiding additional fractures.

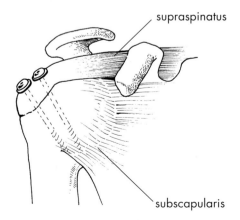

FIGURE 7-4

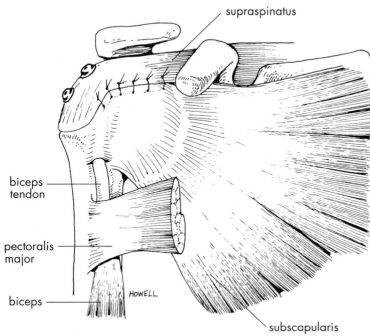

FIGURE 7-5

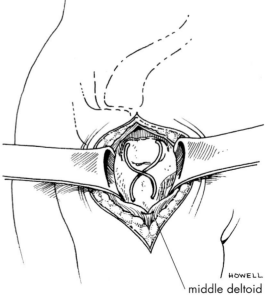

FIGURE 7-6

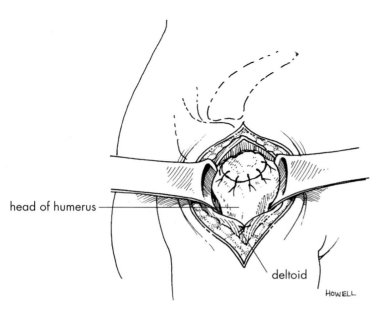

FIGURE 7-7

Closure

Routine closure is performed by allowing the deltoid to reapproximate (see Fig. 7-1) and then repairing the superficial and deep fascial layers. Skin and subcutaneous layers are closed with absorbable suture and a subcuticular stitch, respectively. Steristrips and a light compressive dressing are applied. A drain is unnecessary.

POSTOPERATIVE CARE (SEE CHAPTER 11)

Postoperative care in these patients is tied directly to the quality of bone and to the security of fixation achieved intraoperatively. In younger patients with an intact greater tuberosity, two-screw fixation allows for early full passive motion. In older patients with porotic bone and suture fixation alone, however, the shoulder should be protected and only basic hygiene allowed for the first 2 to 3 weeks. If there is any question as to fracture fixation, pendulum exercises alone are adequate during healing. As soon as callus is evident, with everything clinically moving as a unit, more aggressive physical therapy may be initiated, adding an active component to the rehabilitation process, usually at 4 to 6 weeks.

Strengthening exercises are started at 6 to 8 weeks, with the emphasis on terminal stretching and improving the active and passive range of motion. Patients are instructed that it may take 6 months to achieve a plateau in their improvement. With that in mind, an appropriate goals program may be structured.

Open Reduction of Two-Part Fractures (Surgical Neck)
GENERAL CONSIDERATIONS

This fracture is one of the most common forms of proximal humeral fracture and in many cases is treated conservatively (Fig. 7-8). In an active patient with a two-part displaced Neer fracture, operative reduction and fixation are indicated. In those instances in which displacement is excessive, one may give consideration to various forms of reduction and internal fixation. If there is no apparent proximal extension of the fracture and the head is intact, a locked intramedullary rod may be used. Current models allow one-screw or two-screw proximal head fixation. Distal screws are not often needed because of the tight capture of the rod at the humeral isthmus. The advantage of this system is that it provides rotational and angular control with some fracture compression. Its disadvantage is that it depends on screw fixation for capture of the head fragment. As described previously, the bone in individuals with surgical neck fractures may be very osteoporotic; hence, proximal fixation will be compromised.

Other intramedullary devices exist, such as Rush and Enders rods. These systems, when applied alone, provide angular control and some rotational control with little, if any, fracture compression. The logical addition is the application of tension band wiring. Not only will this add compression, but it will also facilitate rotational control. We believe the ideal form of fixation in these situations is intramedullary rods combined with figure eight tension band wiring, which incorporates the cuff tendons. Figure eight wiring alone, without concomitant intramedullary fixation, should not be used because of the tendency for the fracture to angulate.

AO plate fixation in these fractures has a role in younger patients with good bone stock, but it carries many potential pitfalls, especially in osteoporotic bone. If the plate is applied too proximally, there is a risk of impingement. If applied to the porotic bone of an elderly patient, there is the risk of the plate pulling out and failure of fixation. Screw fixation alone in younger patients with good bone stock may allow the head to be secured to the shaft with certain fracture patterns.

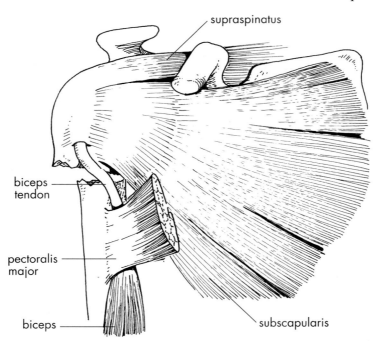

Indications

The technique described is applicable in markedly displaced surgical neck fractures in active, healthy individuals. These fractures are two-part fractures with shaft displacement. Intramedullary fixation should be avoided if there is an associated fracture in the proximal head fragment.

Expectations

Owing to the intact rotator cuff in these individuals, excellent results may be expected. If union takes excessively long and motion is delayed, therapy may take at least 6 months to reach the appropriate result.

SURGICAL TECHNIQUE
Positioning

The "beach chair" position is typically used for intramedullary rodding (see Fig. 2-1) because it allows for a standard anterior deltopectoral approach through which the fracture is directly visualized and reduced. It is important to drape the arm free and have the patient positioned lateral enough so that the arm is over the margin of the table to allow manipulation in all planes.

Approach

For intramedullary rodding with combined figure eight wiring, we use an extended deltopectoral approach (see Fig. 2-23). As the fracture is visualized, if the biceps tendon is trapped at the fracture site, it must first be dislodged to allow reduction. With the fracture reduced, an assessment is made of the proximal exposure. Usually, the rod can be passed from above through the deltopectoral incision (Fig. 7-9). If not, an additional incision, 2 to 3 cm long, is made at the anterolateral corner of the acromion. This incision is taken down to the rotator cuff, which is split longitudinally in the direction of its fibers. A prebent Rush rod is inserted in an antegrade fashion across the fracture site, leaving the proximal portion of the rod a bit prominent. A second Rush rod is placed in similar fashion and left prominent. At this point, a drill hole is made in the lateral aspect of the humeral diaphysis, just distal to the fracture site, and a cerclage wire is passed through it. This wire is brought up beneath the hooked end of the Rush rods (Fig. 7-10). Fracture reduction is confirmed and held.

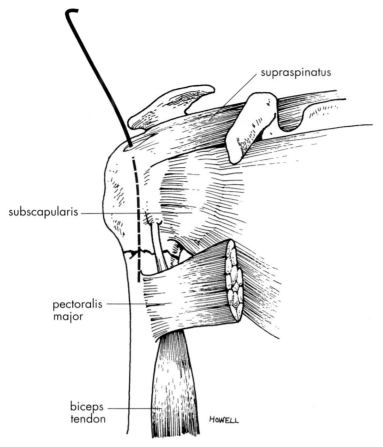

supraspinatus

subscapularis

pectoralis
major

biceps
tendon

HOWELL

FIGURE 7-9

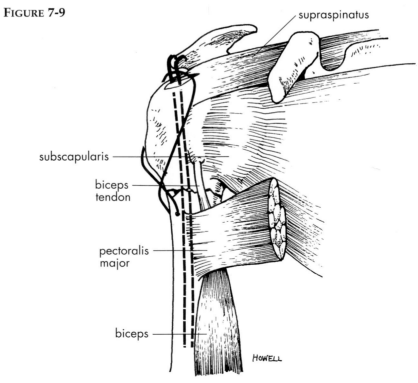

supraspinatus

subscapularis

biceps
tendon

pectoralis
major

biceps

HOWELL

FIGURE 7-10

The cerclage wire is tightened, and the rods are further impacted onto the cerclage wire (Fig. 7-11). Ideally, one would like to have the cerclage wire passed beneath the substance of the rotator cuff, yet through a portion of the greater tuberosity. Obviously, this is difficult to obtain in most cases, and as such the wire and the Rush rod heads will be somewhat prominent. With the fracture stability confirmed by gentle motion of the arm, the rotator cuff interval is reapproximated as much as possible (Fig. 7-12). Sometimes Rush rods alone can provide excellent stability, given the proper fracture configuration. However, optimal stability and fracture compression are best achieved with the combination technique described.

An obvious drawback to the use of Rush rods for the intramedullary component of the fixation is their propensity for backing out during rehabilitation. This would necessitate a second operation. To prevent that problem, many individuals use Enders rods, which have a hole at the proximal portion of the rod through which the cerclage wire may be passed (Fig. 7-13). In this technique, the wire is passed about the greater tuberosity, beneath the rotator cuff, and through the holes in the Enders rods. The rods are then impacted, and the cerclage wire is tightened, reducing the fracture.

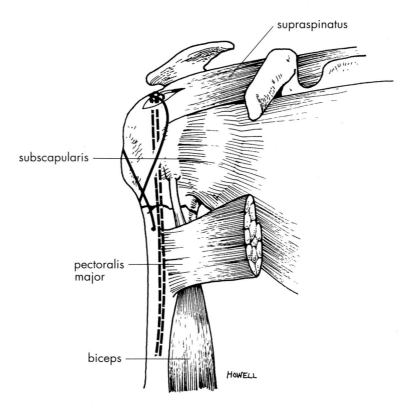

supraspinatus

subscapularis

pectoralis
major

biceps

HOWELL

FIGURE 7-11

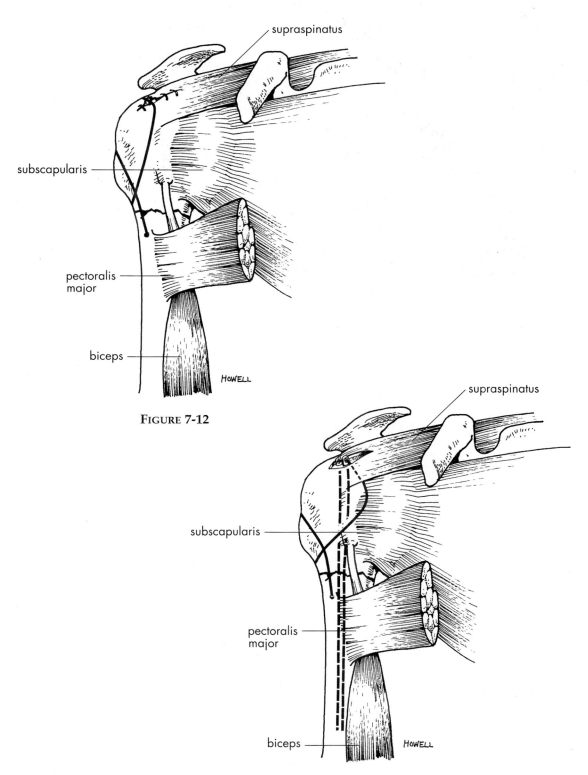

supraspinatus

subscapularis

pectoralis
major

biceps

HOWELL

FIGURE 7-12

supraspinatus

subscapularis

pectoralis
major

biceps

HOWELL

FIGURE 7-13

Following this, the rotator cuff defect may be closed over the Enders rods and cerclage wire (Fig. 7-14).

An alternate technique is the use of a locked intramedullary rod. Fluoroscopic control is helpful. In this approach, a superolateral incision is made in the antero-lateral corner of the acromion (see Fig. 2-35, *b*). The incision is taken down to the deltoid, and a longitudinal split is made in the supraspinatus just medial to the greater tuberosity (Fig. 7-15). A small drill hole is made in the sulcus between the greater tuberosity and the articular surface (Fig. 7-16). A guide wire is placed down the shaft, and the fracture is reduced by either a closed or an open technique (Fig. 7-17). Flexible reamers are used to prepare the canal (Fig. 7-18).

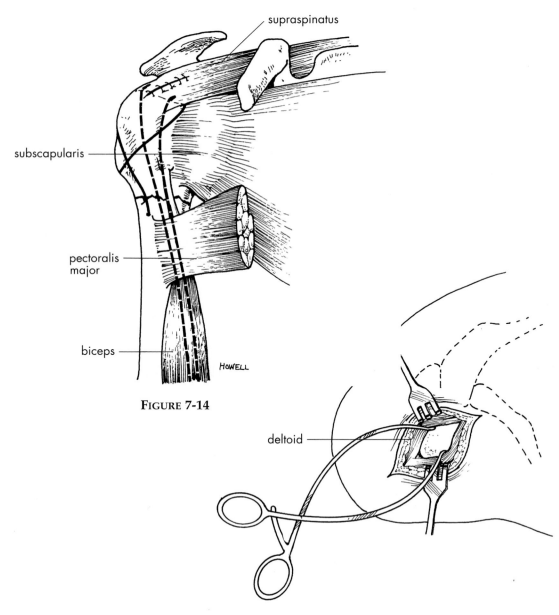

FIGURE 7-14

FIGURE 7-15

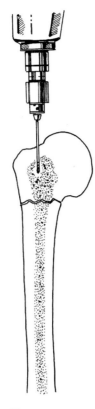

FIGURE 7-16

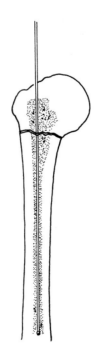

FIGURE 7-17

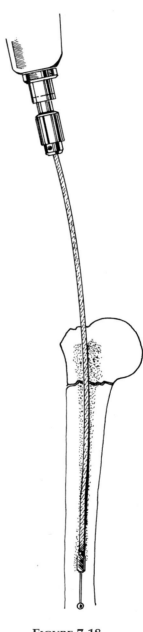

FIGURE 7-18

In most cases of surgical neck fractures, however, canal preparation is not crucial. The smallest rod available will suffice as intramedullary stability is achieved by a 3-point fixation caused by the irregular contours of the humeral shaft and the gentle curve of the humeral rod. If this does not provide adequate stability, distal fixation with a screw(s) may be needed. Next, the impacting device is attached to the rod and inserted over the guide wire (Fig. 7-19). The Biomet rod is unique because it allows both anterior-to-posterior and medial-to-lateral proximal screw fixation. This fixation is ideal in situations of surgical neck fractures because it allows screw placement according to the fracture pattern and size of the proximal fragment. In Fig. 7-20, a screw is placed lateral-to-medial through the rod, capturing the proximal fragment. Seldom will it be necessary to use distal screws with the exception of diaphyseal shaft fractures but, when needed, appropriate dissection and visualization should be used. The distal screws require insertion under direct vision to avoid damage to important neurovascular structures.

Closure

The deltoid falls together, and the subcutaneous and skin layers are closed in the usual fashion. Use of a drain is optional.

POSTOPERATIVE CARE (SEE CHAPTER 11)

Proximal humeral fractures are unique because they require individualized care according to the fracture character, displacement, degree of comminution, and quality of bone. The type of fixation also determines postoperative care. In cases of rigid internal fixation, such as Enders rods with tension band wiring or locked intramedullary rods, passive range of motion may be started on the first postoperative day. In all cases, active motion is avoided for the first 6 weeks until fracture healing is evident. Active exercises are started at 6 weeks and continued until 10 to 12 weeks, at which point, assuming adequate fracture healing and a reasonable range of motion, resistive exercises may be started. It is imperative in the postoperative care of these patients that the surgeon's direction to the therapist be clear. The surgeon must determine fracture stability and the level of healing and from this determination allow therapy to progress or slow down accordingly. Overly exuberant physical therapy early in the recovery may compromise later results. In general, for most fracture patterns, passive motion is continued, using a sling in between exercise periods, for approximately the first 6 weeks. From 6 to 10 weeks, active exercises are performed with terminal stretching. At 10 or 12 weeks, resisted exercises are begun.

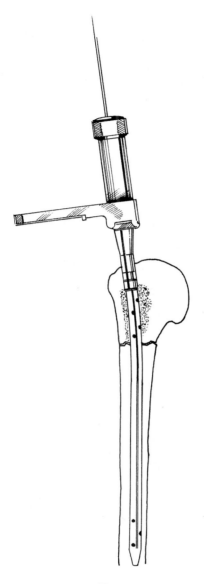

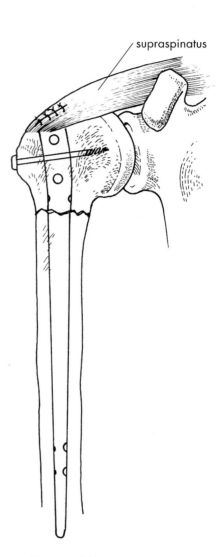

supraspinatus

FIGURE 7-19   **FIGURE 7-20**

Pin Fixation

Another form of fixation is percutaneous pins. These pins may be used to temporarily stabilize surgical neck fractures for the initial 2 to 3 weeks until adequate callus formation occurs. This procedure is performed with the patient in a supine position so that biplane fluoroscopy, imaging both the AP and the axillary planes, may be used. Two experienced surgeons are required—one to reduce and to hold the reduction, and the other to pass the pins. The fracture is manually reduced, and $^{3}/_{16}$-in. pins are then directed antegrade across the fracture from the tuberosity down to the metaphysis (Fig. 7-21, *B*). Sometimes this method of fixation is adequate for sufficient stability to allow fracture healing even though temporary immobilization is required. In two-part surgical neck fractures, we prefer to use two pins from the tuberosity into the shaft. Although it may be difficult, pins may be brought lateral-to-medial retrograde or from anterior-to-posterior in a cephalad fashion to provide cross-pin fixation from shaft-to-head (Fig. 7-21, *A*). These pins are then trimmed, leaving them extending and bent over 1 cm beyond the skin. Betadine ointment is applied, and a sterile dressing is applied to hold the pins in place. Sling immobilization is required for approximately 3 weeks. These pins can be removed easily when callus is evident. The draping technique and sterility aspect are important considerations in percutaneous pin fixation. Absolute sterility is difficult to achieve.

Enders pins and Rush rods can be similarly incorporated for intramedullary fixation in a percutaneous type of arrangement, although often a small incision is required to insert the Enders pins or Rush rods.

POSTOPERATIVE CARE (SEE CHAPTER 11)

In contrast to the previous forms of fixation, percutaneous pin fixation requires sling immobilization until the pins are removed at 3 weeks. The pins can be removed in the office. Following pin removal, passive motion is started. Active motion begins at approximately 6 weeks, followed by resisted exercises at 10 weeks.

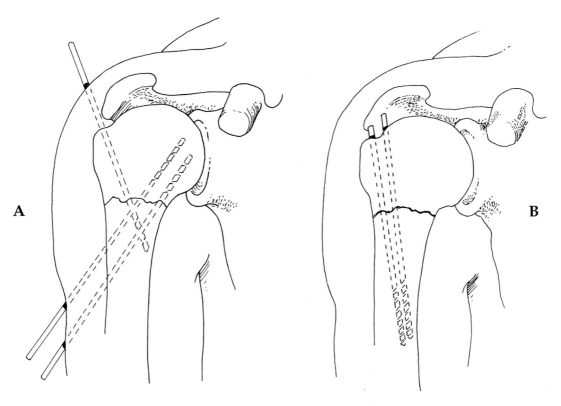

FIGURE 7-21

Plate and Screw Fixation

The use of a plate and screws in fixation of proximal humeral fractures should be limited to those individuals with good quality bone stock. In elderly patients who have advanced osteoporosis, the likelihood of fixation failure (Fig. 7-22) increases. In these patients, intramedullary devices and/or sutures and wires that incorporate the soft tissues in the repair are most successful. In younger patients whose growth plates are closed, plate and screw fixation can achieve rigid internal fixation, allowing early mobilization. Surgical neck fractures and oblique proximal metaphyseal fractures are the most ideal for such fixation. As fracture pattern complexity increases and one starts dealing with displaced and/or fragmented greater or lesser tuberosities, not only does bone quality decrease but secure fixation with a plate is less likely.

A deltopectoral approach is ideally suited to application of plates for proximal humeral fractures (see Fig. 2-23). Because of the required exposure of the humeral shaft, an extended deltopectoral approach is usually necessary and will allow adequate exposure. The plate is ideally positioned on the lateral or tension side of the humerus in the case of surgical neck fractures (Fig. 7-23). L-shaped or T-shaped buttress plates should be used to allow 2 or 3 cancellous screws to be placed in the proximal head fragment. Avoid superior placement of the plate, which may result in later impingement (Fig. 7-24). At least 6 cortices distally are necessary to achieve adequate fixation.

POSTOPERATIVE CARE (SEE CHAPTER 11)

In young patients who have undergone rigid internal fixation, fracture stability should be excellent and immediate passive motion can be used. Depending on the age of the patient and the rate at which the fracture heals, active motion should begin at 6 weeks when healing is evident. Resistive exercises are started at 10 weeks.

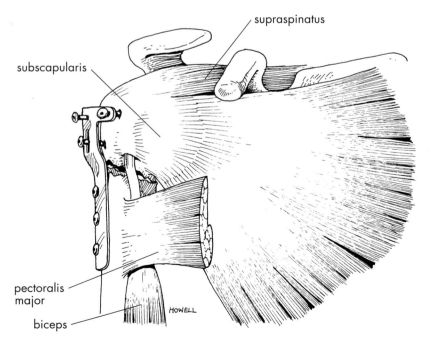

supraspinatus

subscapularis

pectoralis major

biceps

HOWELL

FIGURE 7-22

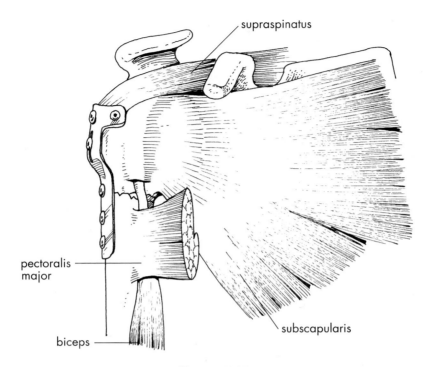

FIGURE 7-23

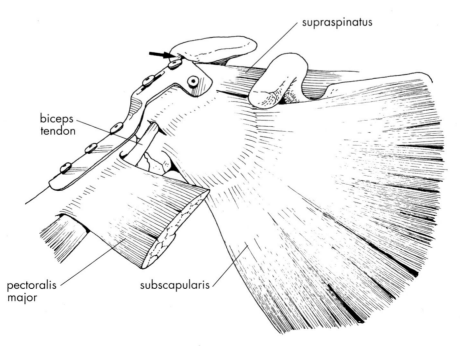

FIGURE 7-24

Surgical Treatment of Three-Part Fractures
GENERAL CONSIDERATIONS

By definition, a three-part fracture consists of a displaced surgical neck fracture, a disimpacted and rotated head, usually with lesser tuberosity attached, and a displaced greater tuberosity (Fig. 7-25). Although several forms of fixation are available for these fractures, our experience with the figure eight wiring has been very successful. This technique incorporates the healthy rotator cuff tissue in the repair, thus avoiding pure bony fixation, which is associated with higher failure rates as seen in the application of plate and screws.

Indications

The indication for open reduction and internal fixation of a three-part fracture is a healthy, active individual. Because of the severity of this injury, it is important to document the preoperative neurological status because occasionally there is an associated axillary neuropathy or plexopathy.

Expectations

With an intact humeral head and one tuberosity in place, the results with three-part fractures can be very satisfactory. It may take 6 months before a satisfactory outcome will be reached in the patient's progress. The patient must understand this process and the goals of the program. A mild loss of end range of motion, especially forward elevation, can be expected but is seldom significant.

SURGICAL TECHNIQUE
Positioning

A "beach chair" position is used, with the arm draped free (see Fig. 2-1). The semi-sitting position may be used (see Fig. 2-2). A half-liter IV bag or inflatable pillow is placed under the ipsilateral scapula, and the shoulder is brought out to and slightly over the edge of the table. This position will allow access to the humeral head. Impervious drapes are used to block out the head and axilla.

Approach

The fracture is exposed through an extended deltopectoral incision (see Fig. 2-23). If a rare concomitant locked anterior dislocation is present, it may be necessary to detach the coracoid process for exposure of the anteroinferior structures. The biceps tendon is used as a landmark for fracture identification, remembering that it lies between the greater and lesser tuberosities (Fig. 7-25).

Procedure

The greater tuberosity will be displaced superiorly and posteriorly. Tag sutures are placed into this. Bringing the greater tuberosity anteriorly and distally and rotating the humeral head internally will reduce the fracture. The head is then reduced to the humeral shaft.

Next, a 14-gauge colpotomy or Dingman needle is placed from the supraspinatus through the greater tuberosity across the head into the lesser tuberosity and out the subscapularis tendon (Fig. 7-26).

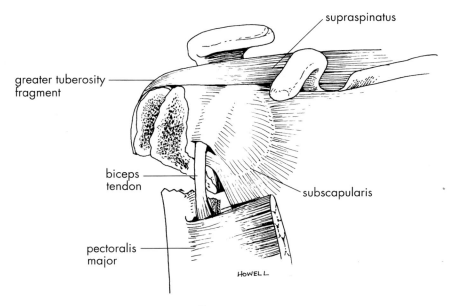

greater tuberosity
fragment

supraspinatus

biceps
tendon

subscapularis

pectoralis
major

HOWELL

FIGURE 7-25

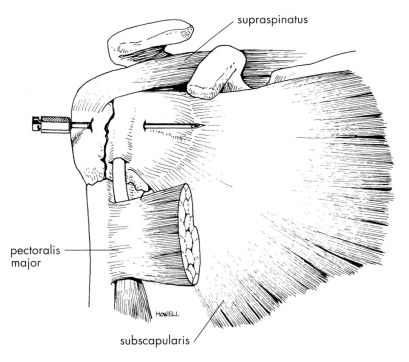

supraspinatus

pectoralis
major

subscapularis

HOWELL

FIGURE 7-26

It is crucial to the success of this procedure that the wire or suture treatment incorporate the tendinous soft tissue of the supraspinatus and subscapularis. Often, these individuals are osteoporotic, and a repair based solely on bony fixation in the head is at risk of failure. In applying this tension band, either wire or heavy nonabsorbable suture material is passed through the colpotomy needle trochar. In our opinion, wire cinches down the fracture more securely than sutures. To achieve optimal position of this trochar, it must be passed through the skin and deltoid into the greater tuberosity and out through the lesser tuberosity. This trochar will allow the passage of the suture or wire. Alternative instruments for passing are a Dingman needle or a Thaires needle. As an alternative, a No. 5 nonabsorbable Mersilene suture may be used. The large curved needle prevents the need for the colpotomy trochar. However, the needle is more difficult to pass and pull through and may not achieve optimal positioning of the wire.

Drill holes are now made in the proximal humeral shaft to accept the placement of the wire or suture distally (Fig. 7-27). The ideal location for drill holes for a tension band principle generally turns out to be on either side of the biceps tendon. In this situation, the biceps often becomes incorporated under the wires, something seemingly unavoidable. Once all sutures are placed, they are tied and the fracture stability is confirmed (Fig. 7-28). The rotator cuff interval and defect are repaired with multiple nonabsorbable sutures (Fig. 7-29).

Closure

The deltoid is allowed to fall back together (see Fig. 2-24) and its superficial fascial layer loosely reapproximated. If excessive bleeding has been encountered intraoperatively, a suction drain may be used for the first 24 hours. A layered closure of the subcutaneous and skin layers is then performed, and a simple Velpeau immobilization is applied.

POSTOPERATIVE CARE (SEE CHAPTER 11)

When physical therapy is started depends on the stability of the fracture fixation. Proper stabilization should provide a stable fracture construct. Thus, in the majority of the cases, passive range of motion may be started immediately. If, however, stability is questionable, delay even passive motion at least 2 to 4 weeks. Radiographical evidence of callus formation will usually be evident at this time. Active exercises are started at 6 weeks when the fracture should be healed. Resistive exercises are started at 10 weeks.

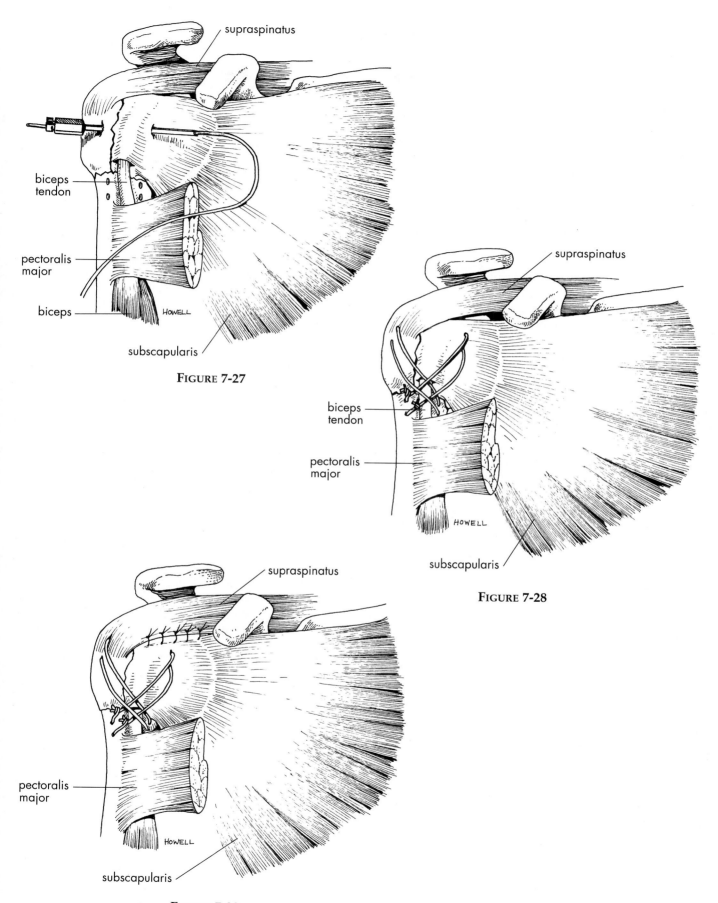

supraspinatus

biceps
tendon

pectoralis
major

biceps

HOWELL

subscapularis

FIGURE 7-27

supraspinatus

biceps
tendon

pectoralis
major

HOWELL

subscapularis

FIGURE 7-28

supraspinatus

pectoralis
major

HOWELL

subscapularis

FIGURE 7-29

Operative Treatment of Four-Part Fractures
GENERAL CONSIDERATIONS

Four-part fractures are rare. When they are identified, the surgeon should look for an associated head dislocation. The head fragment may cause neurovascular embarrassment and necessitate earlier intervention. In most cases, these fractures will require a hemiarthroplasty with careful reattachment of the tuberosities and cuff to the shaft. In younger individuals, consideration may be given to open reduction and internal fixation, realizing the risk of avascular necrosis that may be expected in these fractures. The rare valgus impacted four-part fracture may carry a better prognosis regarding avascular necrosis than the regular four-part fracture. Therefore, this fracture may be more amenable to open reduction and internal fixation than to hemiarthroplasty, which is usually preferable. Open reduction and internal fixation can be done with a combination of straight wires, screws, sutures, and cerclage techniques.

Indications

A hemiarthroplasty is one of the more common options in healthy, active individuals with true four-part fractures. Associated head dislocation may be a relative indication for immediate hemiarthroplasty owing to the high rate of avascular necrosis and malunion as well as to the potential for neurovascular compromise.

Expectations

The patient's expectations following this procedure are guarded. Ideally, one may achieve a functional level of activity above the horizontal. However, because of the occasional inability to achieve union of the tuberosities to the shaft, ultimate range of active motion and function may be limited.

SURGICAL TECHNIQUE
Positioning

A "beach chair" position is used, with the patient's shoulder resting off the side of the table (see Fig. 2-1). The semi-sitting position may also be used (see Fig. 2-2). An inflatable pillow or 500-cc IV bag is placed under the ipsilateral shoulder to bring it into a more advantageous position for the approach. This position will allow access to the humeral shaft for canal preparation during hemiarthroplasty.

Approach

Using an extended deltopectoral incision (see Fig. 2-23), the biceps tendon is identified and the fracture site is exposed (Fig. 7-30). Tag sutures are placed into each of the major bone fragments of the greater and lesser tuberosities. Attached to the greater tuberosity are the supraspinatus and infraspinatus tendons. Mild fragmentation may occur. In this case, multiple tag sutures are helpful, which will help to deliver the greater tuberosity from its position posterior to the humeral head. Similarly, the lesser tuberosity with attached subscapularis is tagged and drawn from its position inferior to the coracoid process.

Procedure

Removal of the free head fragment may not be as easy a task as anticipated. In many cases of fracture dislocation, the head fragment will be markedly displaced posterior to the glenoid or anteriorly in a subcoracoid position. By previously identifying and mobilizing the tuberosity fragments, they can be brought into a position that allows the surgeon better access to the head fragment. By applying gentle traction on the arm, digital manipulation is usually all that is necessary to deliver the head fragment. This fragment is saved for possible bone graft. The humeral shaft is delivered from the wound by gentle extension of the arm and digital pressure from the posterior aspect of the shoulder. Its proximal portion is exposed and any interposed soft tissue is removed. If there is a large proximal extension to the diaphyseal fracture, it should be retained and may be cerclaged to hold it in position.

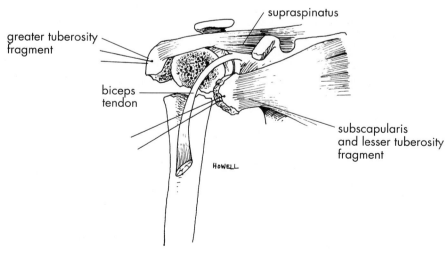

FIGURE 7-30

Preparation of the humeral canal and placement of the prosthesis is one of the more important parts of the procedure and contains several potential technical pitfalls. First, the humeral canal is reamed and broached to accept an appropriate sized humeral stem. Ideally, the broaching should take place with the arm in an appropriate degree of version to accommodate the ultimate prosthesis placement. With the loss of metaphyseal bone from the tuberosity fractures and the accompanying degree of comminution that may be present, the use of cement is required. Using cement will allow control of rotation and a degree of "proudness" of the humeral component. Appropriate version of the humeral component is 30° to 40° of retroversion. In placing the humeral component, remember that metaphyseal bone has been lost and, as such, the component should be placed a bit "proud" relative to the remaining shaft. A trial reduction should leave the flange of the humeral component exposed (at least one hole of the flange of the prosthesis) and the head sitting in an appropriate position relative to the glenoid (Fig. 7-31, A). Fig. 7-31, B shows the head placed too far inferior, which will allow inferior subluxation and poor dynamic cuff control. Note in Fig. 7-31, A that the ideal position places the head opposite the glenoid cavity. The surgeon should be able to place one finger beneath the undersurface of the acromion and the prominence of the greater tuberosity. This step should be confirmed during trial reduction to ensure appropriate positioning of the prosthesis. Mobilization of the tuberosities must be beyond the head and with the capability of being fixed to the shaft.

Because of the loss of proximal bone and the difficulty controlling rotation, a guide to humeral rotation is the bicipital groove. If the prosthesis is placed with the lateral flange just lateral and posterior to the bicipital groove, the appropriate degree of retroversion will be achieved. Fig. 7-32 shows the prosthesis placed at 30° to 40° of retroversion with the arm held in a neutral position. Notice that the flange of the prosthesis rests just posterolateral to the bicipital groove. (See Fig. 5-5, B, which shows the position of the arm at 35° to 40° of external rotation. Note the epicondyles of the elbow, which help confirm appropriate version.)

At this point, the trial humeral component is removed and drill holes are made on each side of the biceps in the humeral shaft to accept two sutures (Fig. 7-32, A). These sutures should be placed before cementation and insertion of the humeral component. Several different sutures may be used, such as a No. 5 Mersilene or Tevdek, which should be strong and nonabsorbable. The humeral canal is prepared as described above, using an appropriate cement technique. The component is secured, incorporating the predetermined degree of retroversion and humeral head height.

The tuberosities are now delivered from the wound, and additional sutures are placed through the lesser and the greater tuberosities. Some surgeons prefer to put one of the sutures through one of the flanges of the prosthesis to allow more security of fixation (Fig. 7-32, B). This, however, is often unnecessary as the goal is to fix the tuberosities and get them to heal to the shaft. We, therefore, do not incorporate the holes of the prosthesis, but bypass the prosthesis, going directly to the shaft (Fig. 7-32, A). These sutures must incorporate the tendinous tissue of the subscapularis and supraspinatus and not rely solely on the porotic bone.

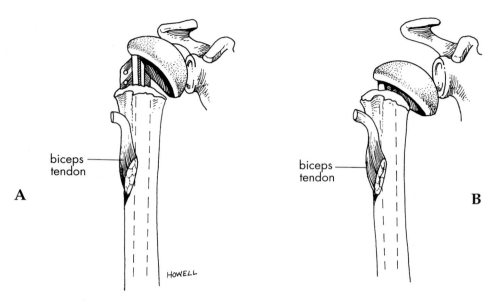

FIGURE 7-31

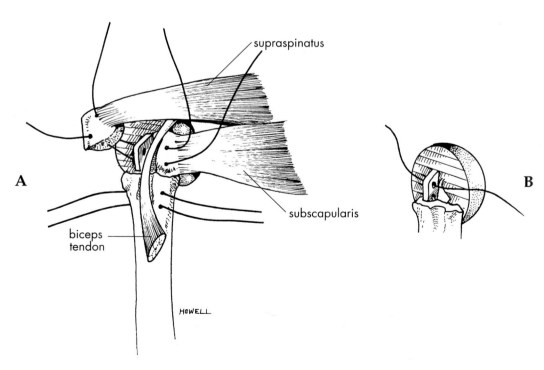

FIGURE 7-32

Before the tuberosities are sutured, their position and their fit are checked, relative to the prosthesis and their resulting prominence. Bone graft is placed under the tuberosities to encourage healing. We also place some bone graft adjacent to the lateral cortex of the humeral shaft to promote healing between the tuberosities and the shaft. In Fig. 7-33, the tuberosities have been brought down into a reduced position, and the two sutures that are holding the tuberosities together have been tied. Note that the sutures are placed under the biceps tendon, thus avoiding a tenodesis. When tenodesis is unavoidable, the sutures must be placed across the tendon. In that case, additional sutures incorporating the tendon into the rotator cuff repair will ensure an appropriate tenodesis.

With the tuberosities sutured together, the next step is to secure the tuberosities to the humeral shaft to promote union and a stable construct for the rotator cuff. This is the critical part of the operation, because if union of the tuberosities to the shaft is not obtained, the procedure will fail and the functional outcome will be poor. The previously placed sutures in the humeral shaft are brought up and placed through the tuberosities, reproducing the technique described for the tuberosity fixation with the exception that no sutures are placed through the flange (Fig. 7-34). The ideal position for these sutures is superior on the tuberosities to incorporate additional tendinous material. These sutures are passed in figure eight fashion, brought back under the biceps tendon, and tightened. The final step is to repair the rotator cuff interval defect. Finally, the shoulder is placed through a gentle range of motion to confirm stability.

Closure

The deltoid is allowed to reapproximate, and its interval is sutured with multiple absorbable sutures. A drain may be a useful adjunct in these cases because of the large amount of exposed cancellous bone and associated bleeding. The subcutaneous and subcuticular layers are closed with absorbable sutures, and Velpeau immobilization is applied.

POSTOPERATIVE CARE (SEE CHAPTER 11)

If stability of the fracture was considered adequate intraoperatively, gentle passive range of motion exercises can be started immediately. These exercises continue for the first 6 weeks, after which time, assuming adequate healing of tuberosities to the shaft, active motion may be started. It is crucial to achieve tuberosity to shaft union for success. Resistive exercises are added at 10 to 12 weeks. It is important to have the patient understand that this physical therapy program may last 6 to 12 months to achieve the optimal result.

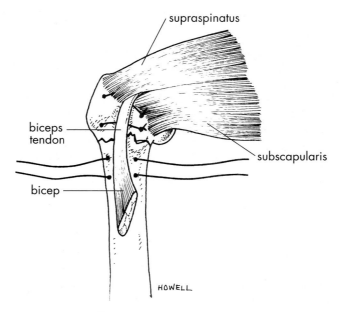

FIGURE 7-33

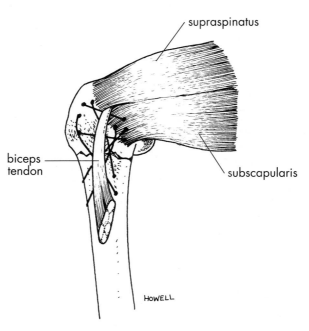

FIGURE 7-34

Operative Treatment of Scapular Fractures

GENERAL CONSIDERATIONS

The majority of scapular fractures require only sling immobilization and early rehabilitation. Body fractures that are more significantly displaced may be immobilized in a sling for 3 weeks, followed by passive motion with anticipated good results. Glenoid fossa fractures that are displaced or angulated, especially if associated with humeral head dislocation, should be considered for operative reduction with internal fixation. Fracture dislocations of the glenoid with significantly large and displaced fractures of the glenoid rim should also undergo operative reduction. Preoperative evaluation with CT scanning, tomography, or both is helpful to define the fracture pattern and degree of displacement.

SURGICAL TECHNIQUE

Positioning

To allow for both anterior and posterior exposure, the patient is placed in a lateral decubitus position with the involved shoulder up (see Fig. 2-4). The prone position is preferred by some surgeons (see Fig. 2-3) but obviously precludes a combined anterior-posterior approach. An IV bag or axillary roll is placed under the down side axilla. The arm is draped free.

Approach

The skin incision is parallel with the inferior margin of the scapular spine, out laterally as far as the lateral edge of the acromion and extended distally along the medial scapular border to its inferior tip (Fig. 7-35). The deltoid is freed from the underlying infraspinatus and scapular spine and allowed to retract distally. The underlying infraspinatus is elevated from its fossa, beginning at the superomedial corner of the scapula (Fig. 7-36). As this is elevated medially, the underlying suprascapular bundle and its branches are identified (Fig. 7-37).

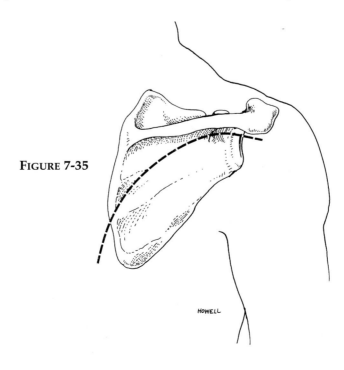

FIGURE 7-35

HOWELL

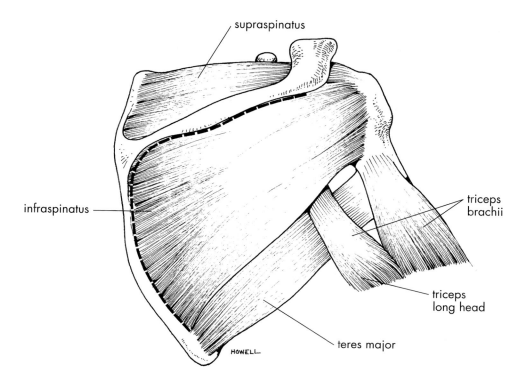

FIGURE 7-36

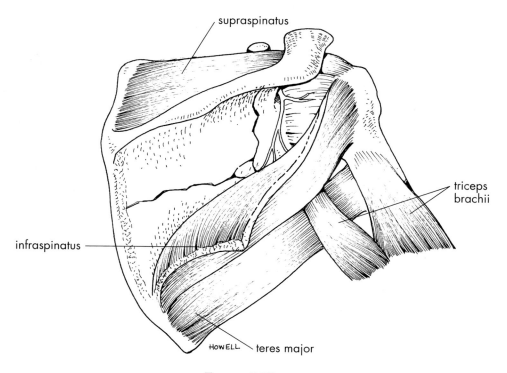

FIGURE 7-37

The surgeon must exercise caution to avoid injury to the principal branch of the suprascapular nerve, rounding the spinoglenoid notch at the base of the scapular spine medially. With the infraspinatus elevated, AO fixation may be readily applied. Note in Figs. 7-38 and 7-39 that the plates are best applied to the margins of the scapular body because of the thicker cortical bone—in this case the medial border of the scapula and the juncture of the scapular spine with the body of the scapula. Often, fixation of body segments, particularly the lateral column, reduces any intraarticular glenoid fractures.

An alternative approach for glenoid face and neck fractures is a split between the inferior margin of the infraspinatus and the superior border of the teres minor (Fig. 7-40). Using this approach, one may use a vertical incision as for posterior instability (see Fig. 2-4). The infraspinatus and teres minor are exposed after elevating the deltoid (Fig. 7-41).

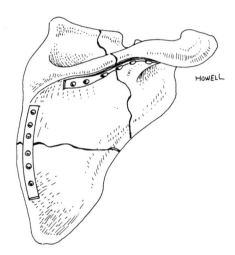

FIGURE 7-38

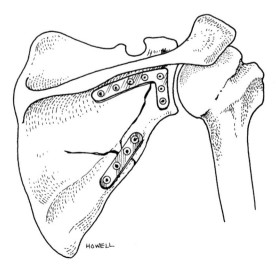

FIGURE 7-39

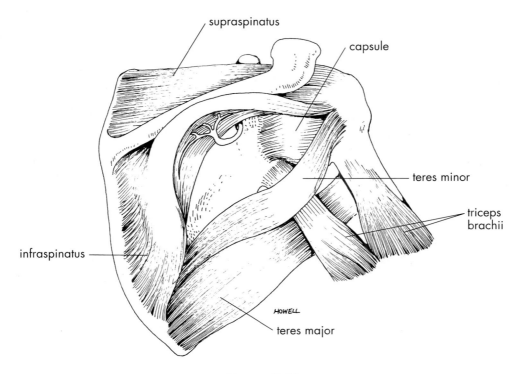

FIGURE 7-40

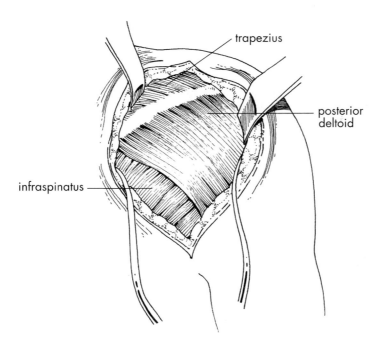

FIGURE 7-41

This exposure has several advantages: it maintains the attachment of the origin and insertion of the infraspinatus, it allows visualization of the suprascapular nerve, and it provides excellent exposure of the joint. With the infraspinatus elevated and the teres minor brought inferiorly, a "T" capsulotomy is made posteriorly to expose the articular surface and the scapular neck (Fig. 7-42). In the case of posterior rim fractures, interfragmentary fixation is usually adequate (Fig. 7-43). Markedly displaced glenoid neck fractures will require more than simply interfragmentary fixation. In these situations a neutralization plate, often in the form of an L-plate running along the scapular spine, will provide appropriate neutralization and stability (Fig. 7-39). Scapular spine fractures often allow the distal fragment to be displaced downwardly, creating impingement if the spine is not reduced and plated.

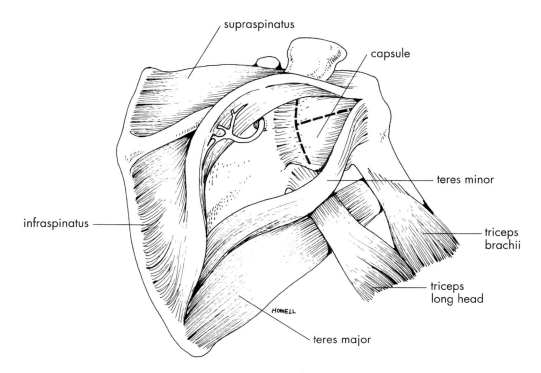

supraspinatus

capsule

infraspinatus

teres minor

triceps brachii

triceps long head

teres major

HOWELL

FIGURE 7-42

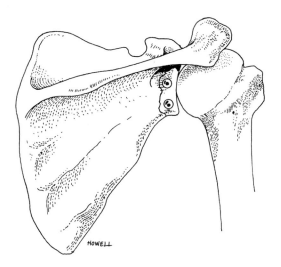

HOWELL

FIGURE 7-43

A final approach to inferior and mid-to-lateral scapular fractures is to incise the skin from the spine of the scapula to the inferior pole of the scapula along the medial border (Fig. 7-44, *A*). The deltoid is incised off the spine and retracted distally (Fig. 7-44, *B*). The infraspinatus is then elevated from the inferior pole all the way up to the spinoglenoid notch, identified by visualization of the suprascapular nerve coursing into its undersurface (Fig. 7-44, *C*). The capsule can be entered, if desired, at the level of the glenohumeral joint (Fig. 7-44). Usually, plating and screws are appropriate treatment for fixation.

Anteroinferior glenoid fractures are approached from the front through a deltopectoral incision. The joint is then entered, and the fracture is fixed from the inside or fixed from above with a lag principle. This is a difficult approach because of the medial neurovascular structures, particularly when fixation is attempted from inferiorly or from medially into the glenoid face.

Closure

Closure is obtained by reapproximating the capsule. The infraspinatus is secured to the superomedial edge of the scapular spine and the medial scapular border. The deltoid is similarly repaired to the bone of the scapular spine. If a splitting approach has been used for the deltoid, infraspinatus, and teres minor, they simply fall together. The patient is placed into sling immobilization. However, a shoulder spica may be necessary in more comminuted fractures or less compliant patients.

POSTOPERATIVE CARE (SEE CHAPTER 11)

Protective immobilization is worn for 3 to 6 weeks. Patients can begin passive assisted motion out of the support during the first week as pain allows. Active motion begins at 3 weeks and progresses to resisted exercises at 6 weeks.

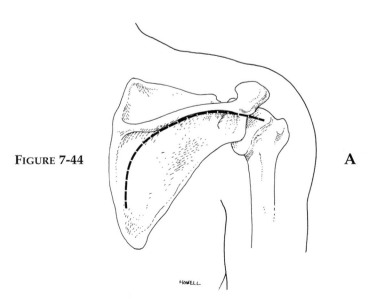

FIGURE 7-44

A

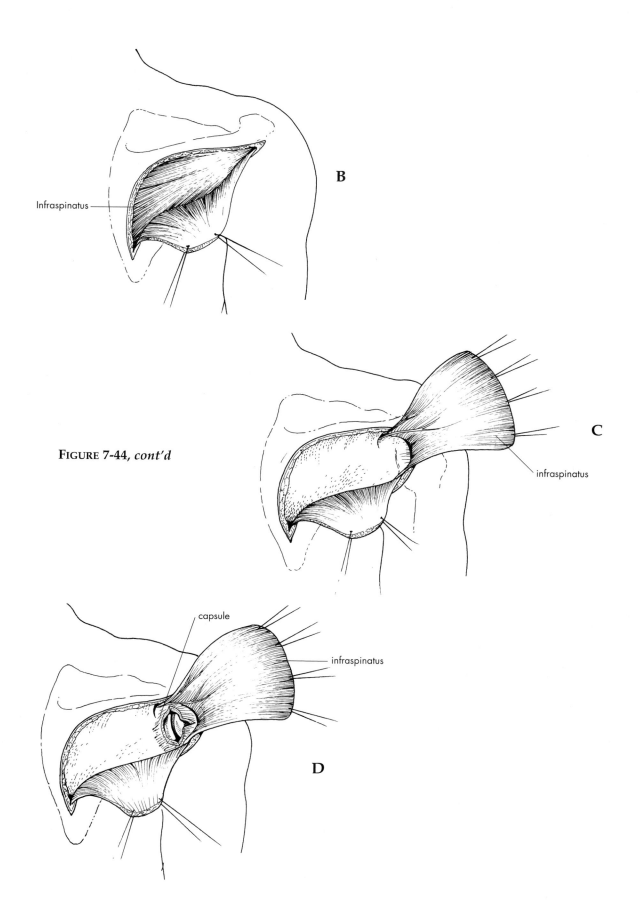

Infraspinatus

B

FIGURE 7-44, *cont'd*

infraspinatus

C

capsule

infraspinatus

D

Operative Treatment of Clavicular Fractures
GENERAL CONSIDERATIONS

Clavicle fractures are classified according to location. Type I fractures involve the diaphyseal midshaft portion of the clavicle and have a high union rate (Fig. 7-45). Type II fractures are more lateral and are classified as A, B, or C, according to their location relative to the coracoclavicular ligaments. A Type IIA fracture is just medial to the coracoclavicular ligaments (Fig. 7-46). Because of the loss of coracoclavicular stability, the medial fragment becomes unstable and displaces superiorly, which results in greater risk of nonunion in this type of fracture. However, with or without union, these fractures tend to have good functional outcomes. A Type IIB fracture involves a fracture within the ligaments or just lateral to them, thus making it a stable fracture (Fig. 7-47). Type IIC is an intraarticular fracture at the acromioclavicular joint (Fig. 7-48). Type III fractures are seldom seen and involve the medial end of the clavicle near the sternoclavicular articulation (Fig. 7-49).

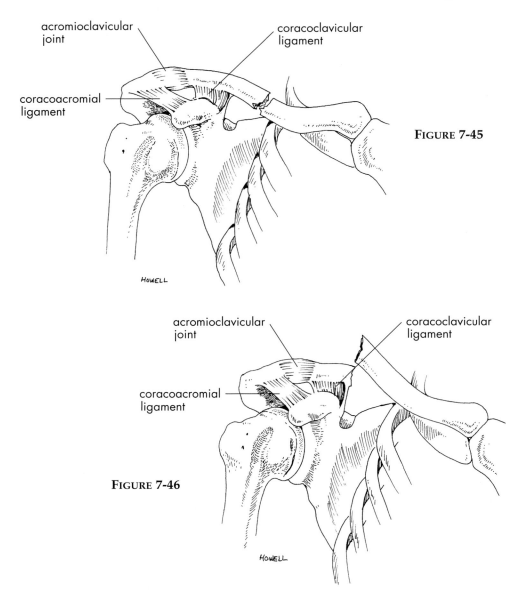

FIGURE 7-45

FIGURE 7-46

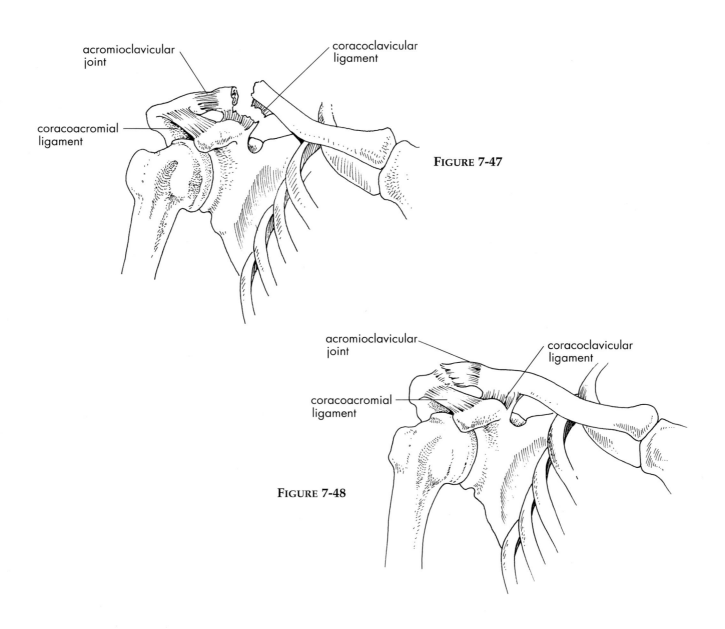

acromioclavicular joint

coracoclavicular ligament

coracoacromial ligament

FIGURE 7-47

acromioclavicular joint

coracoclavicular ligament

coracoacromial ligament

FIGURE 7-48

acromioclavicular joint

coracoclavicular ligament

coracoacromial ligament

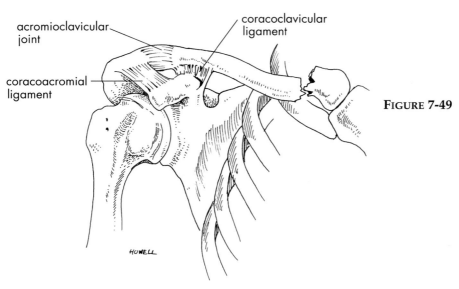

FIGURE 7-49

HOWELL

Indications

The majority of clavicular fractures may be treated conservatively with anticipation of union and a good functional return. However, there are instances when internal fixation may be necessary: (1) fractures at or near the acromioclavicular joint with concomitant disruption of the coracoclavicular ligaments, (2) severely displaced Type I midshaft or Type IIA (see Fig. 7-22) fractures with resulting tenting of the skin and poor cosmesis, (3) fractures with associated vascular injury that would require exposure of the underlying vascular structures before repair, and (4) clavicular nonunions.

Typically, a 3.5 AO reconstruction plate or some form of threaded intramedullary fixation are the most appropriate forms of fixation. In Type II injuries, occasionally the outer clavicular segment is small and comminuted and can be excised and the clavicle can be fixed to the coracoid as in a Weaver-Dunn procedure, perhaps with some additional internal fixation. AO plates are malleable, allowing them to be contoured to the curved shape of the clavicle. In contrast, intramedullary devices, by their nature, avoid the irregular exterior of the clavicle, achieving their stability internally by three-point fixation. Smooth pins should be avoided because of the risk of migration. The more lateral the fracture in routine clavicular shaft fractures, the better the application for intramedullary fixation. In general, for clavicular fractures, plate fixation is more easily accomplished. In a Type II outer clavicular fracture, a plate can be used if four secure cortices can be positioned in the lateral fragment. With such surgery for Type II outer clavicular fractures, we encourage two procedures: (1) after plate or intramedullary fixation or (2) additional fixation of coracoid to clavicle.

Expectations

A stable, painless, healed fracture may be expected. Hardware may be a problem, especially plates, and may require subsequent removal. There is also a question as to whether open reduction and internal fixation produce a higher nonunion rate. Type II distal clavicle fractures may develop some acromioclavicular joint pain, but will seldom necessitate a Mumford procedure. Type II fractures of the clavicle often lead to nonunion if treated nonsurgically.

SURGICAL TECHNIQUE
Positioning

The "beach chair" position (see Fig. 2-1) is used with additional padding under the involved scapula to elevate the shoulder, allowing access to both the anterior and the superior aspects of the clavicle. A special headrest is available, such as a McConnell, allowing better access to the superior aspect of the shoulder, much as in the semi-sitting position (see Fig. 2-2).

Approach

Displaced midshaft fractures are exposed using a curvilinear incision 1 cm anterior and therefore inferior to the clavicle (Fig. 7-50). This is taken down through subcutaneous tissue to the platysma and trapezial fascia.

The fracture is subperiosteally exposed and reduced. Standard AO technique is used to achieve fixation. A 3.5-mm reconstruction plate is used, allowing contouring to the clavicular shape (Fig. 7-51). Extreme care is necessary to avoid the neurovascular structures inferior and posterior to the clavicle, especially during the drilling and the determination of screw length.

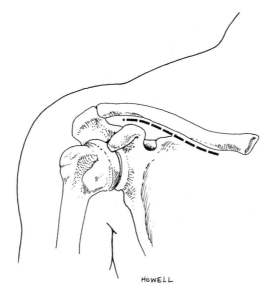

HOWELL

FIGURE 7-50

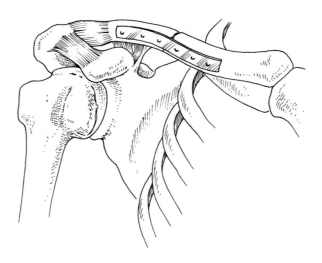

FIGURE 7-51

To avoid injury to these structures, the plate is ideally placed on the anteroinferior aspect of the clavicle, if fracture orientation allows. This will allow the direction of the drill tap and screw to be from anteroinferior to posterosuperior, providing the least opportunity for neurovascular compromise. It is acceptable, should the situation dictate, to place the plate superiorly.

If intramedullary fixation is used, a similar but shorter incision is made and the fracture is exposed. The lateral or distal fragment is elevated, exposing its medullary canal. A guide wire is then placed from the fracture toward the acromioclavicular joint retrograde, exiting at the posterior wall of the lateral fragment (Fig. 7-52). The fracture is reduced and held in place while the guide wire is passed antegrade, back across the fracture, to an appropriate depth. With the guide wire in place, a cannulated screw may be inserted across the guide wire to an appropriate depth. Alternative forms of intramedullary fixation consist of Knowles, Steinmann, or Rockwood pins. In each of these situations, the pin itself is brought back from the fracture site and then, with the fracture reduced, is drilled into the medial clavicular fragment. All of these fixation devices have a threaded shaft and, as such, resist migration. The cannulated screw and the Knowles and Rockwood pins will further resist medial migration with their nuts.

Once the fracture has been stabilized with the fixation device, the screw is left just within the subcutaneous tissue so that it can be removed later once union has been achieved. If they are not needed, the nut and screw should not be used since they may cause significant irritation under the skin.

POSTOPERATIVE CARE (SEE CHAPTER 11)

It is critical following fixation of such fractures to have temporary immobilization in a sling for 2 to 4 weeks. This immobilization is especially critical with intramedullary fixation and especially applicable to fractures of the outer clavicle, such as Type II fractures. Occasionally, passive motion may be started immediately below horizontal. Active motion is usually delayed until callus is present at approximately 5 to 6 weeks. Resisted exercises are delayed for approximately 8 to 10 weeks.

Type II Outer Clavicular Fractures (Neer's Classifications)

A Type II outer clavicular fracture with disruption of the coracoclavicular ligaments frequently causes a significant cosmetic deformity. If surgery is considered, there are three options:

1. A fairly secure malleable plate fixation, only if four cortices can be obtained in the distal fragment (Fig. 7-53, A).
2. Retrograde threaded one-pin or two-pin fixation from lateral to medial into the proximal fragment (Fig. 7-53, B).
3. Excision of the distal fragment and fixation of the clavicle to the coracoid (see Fig. 8-18).
4. Leave fragment in place and fix clavicle to the coracoid (Fig. 7-53, C).

Another option is either plating or threaded pin fixation with fixation of the clavicle to the coracoid. This option would obviously give a belt-and-suspenders secure fixation. We recommend at least two operations in such fractures: plate plus coracoclavicular fixation or threaded pins plus coracoclavicular fixation.

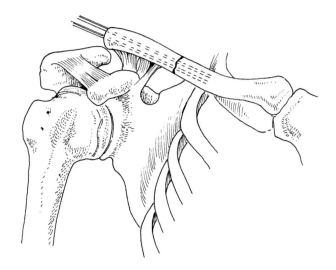

FIGURE 7-52

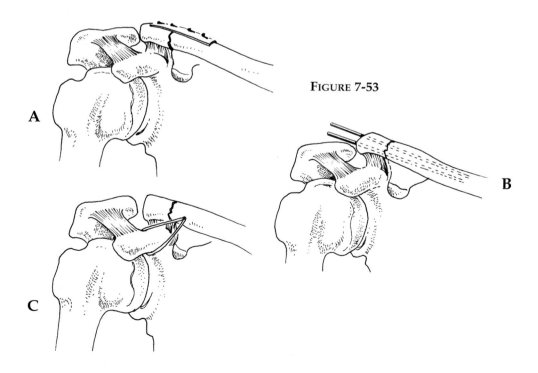

FIGURE 7-53

Late Fracture Problems

Frequently, late fracture problems may lead to the need for greater and lesser tuberosity osteotomies and mobilization. Occasionally, the head also requires osteotomy into a better position. Although this chapter did not deal specifically with these fracture problems and osteotomies, several technical points should be mentioned, particularly regarding the greater tuberosity. It is important to emphasize that the osteotomy cut is started from the lateral shaft up into the undersurface of the displaced greater tuberosity, breaking into the articular surface of the joint itself. The rotator cuff on each side is then mobilized, and the tuberosity is advanced distally. Occasionally, it is necessary to remove some bone from the undersurface of the osteotomy cut to allow more appropriate mobilization of the bone-tendon complex distally. It is then secured in place with either a screw, tension band figure eight fixation, or both. Postoperatively, the arm is immobilized in an abducted position until fully healed, approximately 4 to 6 weeks. Gentle passive motion, followed by active and resisted exercises, can then be started.

Acromioclavicular Joint   8

Introduction

The acromioclavicular joint is involved in several traumatic and degenerative disorders of the shoulder. Arthritis affects this joint in several different forms—the most common is osteoarthritis. Osteoarthritis is typically seen in those patients involved in manual labor or contact sports. The diagnosis is easily made, owing to the classic radiographical changes and physical findings. Pain will be well localized, both by the patient describing its location and by palpation. Pain is seldom referred to in contrast to impingement and rotator cuff problems. Cross-arm adduction and abduction will reproduce the pain. Forward elevation, unlike in patients with rotator cuff or impingement, will not cause as much discomfort. Conservative measures, although providing temporary relief, will prove mainly palliative. As the arthritis progresses, the patient may require an excision of the distal clavicle (Mumford procedure).

In patients with this arthritic process, there is often a concomitant problem with impingement, rotator cuff pathology, or both. If the acromioclavicular joint disease is advanced, the inferior acromial and clavicular spurs may irritate the underlying supraspinatus tendon, causing an associated impingement tendinitis (Fig. 8-1). If the disease is symptomatic enough to require a decompression, attention should also be directed to the osteophytes on the undersurface of the clavicle to provide adequate decompression of the subacromial space (Fig. 8-2). In this circumstance, a resection of the outer clavicle is unusual.

The Zanca view is an AP view relative to the coronal planes of the body performed by directing the tube anteriorly, 10° to 15° cephalad. This view projects the acromioclavicular joint above the scapular spine. To avoid overexposure, the kilovoltage should be decreased. This view allows determination of the degree of arthritis, the presence of inferior acromial or clavicular spurs, and any cystic changes of the distal clavicle.

Another common disorder of the acromioclavicular joint is traumatic separation. Although several classifications for this problem exist, the one most commonly used is that of Rockwood, which describes the displacement of the outer clavicle as the degree of coracoclavicular and acromioclavicular ligamentous injury progresses. (Fig. 8-3). Grade I injuries (Fig. 8-3, *A*) involve only the acromioclavicular joint itself with preservation of the coracoclavicular ligaments. As the injury progresses, the relative involvement of the joint and coracoclavicular ligaments increases to the point where, in Type III injuries (Fig. 8-3, *C*), there is complete disruption of coracoclavicular ligaments, acromioclavicular joint capsule, and ligamentous construct. This results in superior migration.

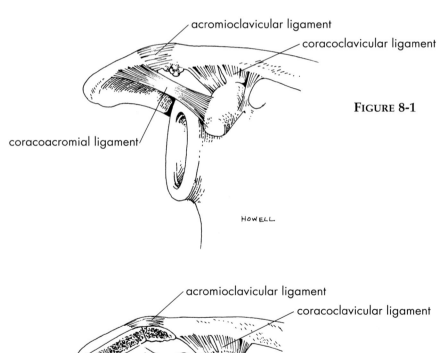

acromioclavicular ligament

coracoclavicular ligament

coracoacromial ligament

HOWELL

FIGURE 8-1

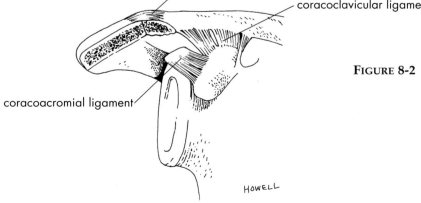

acromioclavicular ligament

coracoclavicular ligament

coracoacromial ligament

HOWELL

FIGURE 8-2

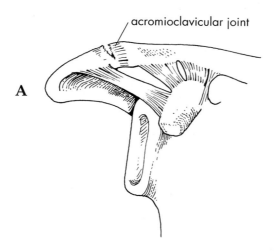

acromioclavicular joint

A

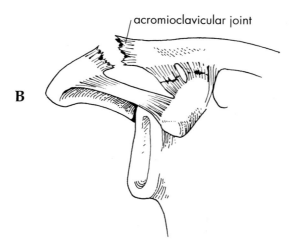

acromioclavicular joint

B

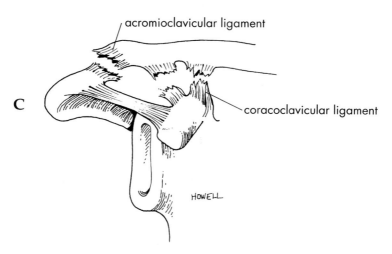

acromioclavicular ligament

coracoclavicular ligament

C

HOWELL

FIGURE 8-3

In Type IV injuries, the force is directed posteriorly with disruption of all ligamentous restraints as in Type III injuries, but with a significant posterior translation of the distal clavicle and buttonholing through the trapezius fascia (Fig. 8-3, *D*). Type V injuries, described as an "ear tickler" because of the marked superior displacement of the clavicle, are caused by buttonholing of the clavicle through the trapezius fascia superiorly (Fig. 8-3, *E*). Type VI injuries are extremely rare, consisting of an inferior dislocation of the clavicle beneath the coracoid (Fig. 8-4). Most surgeons agree that Type I, Type II, and most Type III injuries can be successfully treated conservatively. Types IV, V, and VI may require reconstruction. The decision to operate must be based on several criteria, including injury classification, patient's activity level, degree of displacement, type of work (manual or sedentary), and, in some cases, cosmesis.

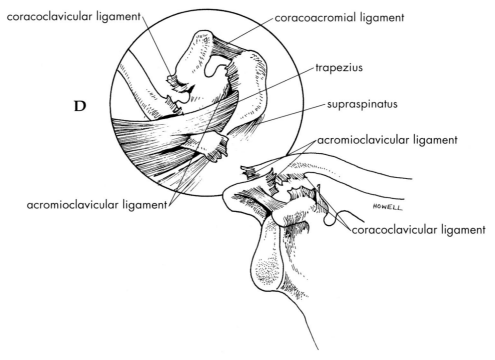

FIGURE 8-3, *cont'd*

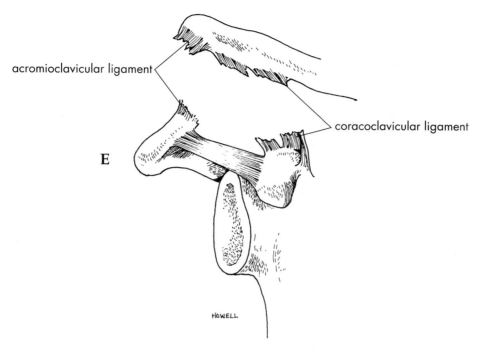

acromioclavicular ligament

coracoclavicular ligament

E

HOWELL

FIGURE 8-3, *cont'd*

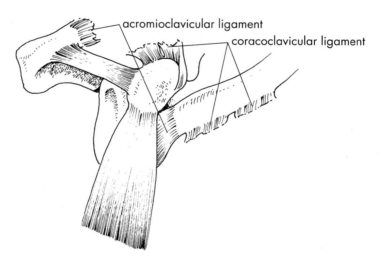

acromioclavicular ligament

coracoclavicular ligament

FIGURE 8-4

Distal Clavicle Resection
GENERAL CONSIDERATIONS

Excision of the distal clavicle is reserved for those individuals with a painful joint refractory to the usual conservative measures and who exhibit radiographical evidence of degenerative arthritis. Intraarticular injections may help confirm the acromioclavicular joint as the etiology of the pain. With this impairment, a simple distal clavicular excision is usually a successful procedure.

Indications

Ideal patients for this procedure are those with isolated acromioclavicular pathology in which associated impingement, cervical disc pathology, rotator cuff tears, and/or instability have been ruled out as possible contributing factors. In most of these patients, the diagnosis is easily made. The physical examination will demonstrate point tenderness over the acromioclavicular joint and pain with forced crossed-arm adduction with the arm internally rotated, thus compressing the joint. There will also be pain with abduction, particularly against resistance in the coronal plane. Typical radiographical findings will include sclerosis and irregularity of the joint surfaces, loss of joint space, cystic erosion, and, in more advanced stages of degenerative arthritis, inferior osteophyte formation. Weightlifters sometimes present with osteolysis and resorption of the distal clavicle.

Often, in cases of acromioclavicular separation, distal clavicle excision is combined with some form of fixation of the clavicle to the coracoid (see Fig. 8-30).

Expectations

More than 90% of these patients obtain pain relief and are able to resume nearly all athletic and work-related endeavors. Late Cybex testing after resection has shown that the shoulder regains normal strength. Occasionally, bench pressing proves challenging.

SURGICAL TECHNIQUE
Positioning

The patient is placed in the "beach chair" position (see Fig. 2-1). It is advantageous to have a headrest or to use the semi-sitting position to allow an approach to the superior aspect of the shoulder (see Fig. 2-2). The arm is draped free following a standard surgical prep. The drapes are carried high onto the neck to allow access to the superior aspect of the shoulder.

Approach

A linear incision is made beginning 1 cm posterior to the acromioclavicular joint, coursing anteriorly and inferiorly 1 cm past the joint (see Figs. 2-36 and 2-37). A horizontal incision may be preferred. Medial and lateral dissection allows exposure of the underlying deltotrapezial fascia. This tissue is incised on top of the clavicle in its midsection from medial to lateral.

Procedure

Subperiosteal dissection exposes the lateral 2 cm of the clavicle and the very medial aspect of the acromial facet (Fig. 8-5, *A*). Retractors are placed anteriorly and posteriorly in a subperiosteal fashion (see Fig. 2-38). A Bristow elevator can be placed into the acromioclavicular joint from lateral to elevate the outer clavicle. Either an osteotome or an oscillating saw is used to excise the clavicle (Fig. 8-5, *B*).

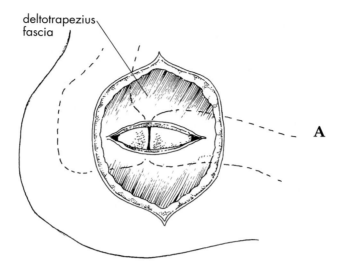

deltotrapezius
fascia

A

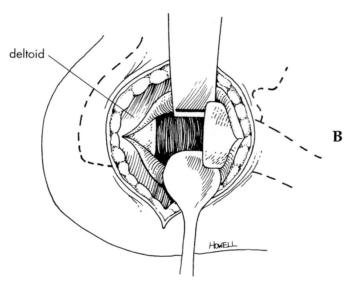

deltoid

B

HOWELL

FIGURE 8-5

This excision is most easily performed by directing the cut from anterior to posterior. Orientation of this cut in both coronal and sagittal planes is important. As shown in Fig. 8-6, approximately 1.5 to 2 cm of the distal clavicle is excised. The vertical orientation of this cut must provide adequate decompression of the joint. As shown in Fig. 8-7, if this cut is too oblique, there is a risk of residual impingement on the superior surface of the clavicle and the acromion. If the cut has appropriate vertical orientation, there will be an adequate decompression of the joint. When viewed from above, the osteotomy is oriented parallel with the articular surface of the acromial facet (Fig. 8-8). If this cut is directed laterally, there will be a convergence of the posterior margin of the clavicle and the posterior aspect of the acromial facet, resulting in residual impingement (Fig. 8-9). The amount of distal clavicle excised should not exceed 2 cm, thus preserving the coracoclavicular ligament attachments. Once the lateral fragment has been excised, the margins of the osteotomy site are palpated and a rongeur is used on the rough edges. If the surgeon's finger does not impinge between the clavicle and the acromion with crossed-arm adduction, enough clavicle has been removed.

Closure

The wound is closed in layers, carefully reapproximating the fascial layers of the deltoid and the trapezius. Deep sutures will help eliminate the dead space. A drain is optional but seldon required with an adequate closure. The subcutaneous and subcuticular layers are closed with absorbable sutures, and Steristrips are applied to the wound.

POSTOPERATIVE CARE (SEE CHAPTER 11)

Because of the minimal disruption of the soft tissue and muscle planes, passive motion is started immediately and active motion is added as pain allows, often at 1 week. Resistive exercises may be started as early as the second or third week with an anticipated return to work and sports at approximately 2 months.

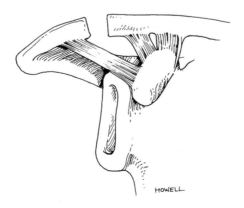

FIGURE 8-6

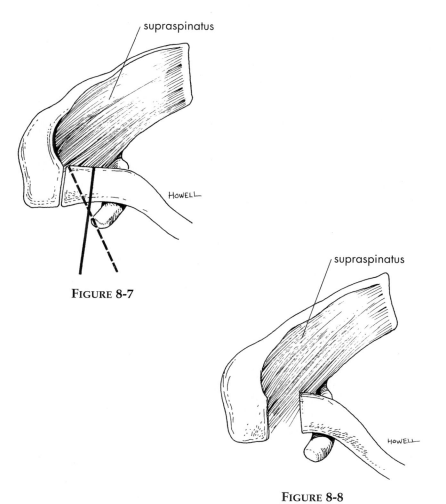

supraspinatus

HOWELL

FIGURE 8-7

supraspinatus

HOWELL

FIGURE 8-8

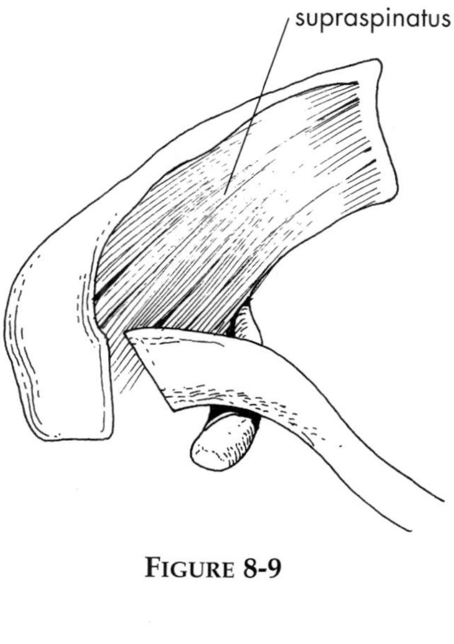

supraspinatus

FIGURE 8-9

Coracoclavicular Reconstruction for Acute and Chronic Separations
GENERAL CONSIDERATIONS

Numerous techniques may be used for coracoclavicular reconstructions. These include isolated pin fixation of the acromioclavicular joint, combination of coracoacromial ligament reconstruction and concomitant pin fixation (Fig. 8-10), cancellous screw stabilization with a ligament reconstruction (Fig. 8-11), coracoacromial ligament transfer to the excised end of the distal clavicle with or without concomitant coracoclavicular stabilization (Fig. 8-12), and, in rare occasions, coracoid transfer (Fig. 8-13).

The specific type of treatment depends on whether the injury is acute or chronic. In chronic acromioclavicular separations, the displaced clavicle has allowed medialization of the scapula, thus making acromioclavicular reduction improbable. In these situations, the distal clavicle should be excised to allow reduction. Reconstruction should not only reduce the clavicle but also provide a restraint to superior clavicular migration. The technique that we often use in the chronic situation is that of a synthetic graft reconstruction of the coracoacromial ligament. The graft consists of nine individual strands of a No. 1 absorbable monofilament suture material, which are then braided. This braid is combined with a coracoacromial ligament transfer after the method of Weaver-Dunn, thus providing an autogenous long-term support system to back up the temporary absorbable graft. The surgeon may also consider autogenous palmaris longus graft if additional autogenous tissues are required for stability. This technique avoids the potential long-term problems associated with permanent fixation devices.

In acute acromioclavicular separations, the joint is usually reducible without need for clavicular excision, and the coracoclavicular ligaments may be reapproximated and repaired. Occasionally, the articular surface may be damaged and may require concomitant excision. Treatment options in acute separations run the gamut from percutaneous closed acromioclavicular joint pinnings to open coracoclavicular screw fixation with concomitant ligament repair, coracoclavicular ligament reconstruction with graft stabilization, and, in some cases, coracoclavicular ligament reconstruction with coracoacromial ligament transfer to the undersurface of the clavicle. Our present approach in acute situations is similar to procedures for chronic separations except that the outer clavicle is not excised. In the Weaver-Dunn method, the coracoacromial ligament is placed through a drill hole and backed up with the braided absorbable suture technique.

Indications

The principal indications for coracoclavicular reconstructions are Grade III separations or greater. All chronic separations should have a concomitant excision of the distal clavicle (see distal clavicle excision, p. 240). Rarely, acute reconstructions may also require resection of the distal clavicle if there is associated damage to the articular surface.

Expectations

The intent of this surgery is to provide a reduction of the displaced clavicle, thus lessening the cosmetic deformity and chronic fatigue that some individuals with Grade III or greater separations experience. In most cases, pain will be minimal and the laborer and athlete may return to their endeavors at approximately 3 months.

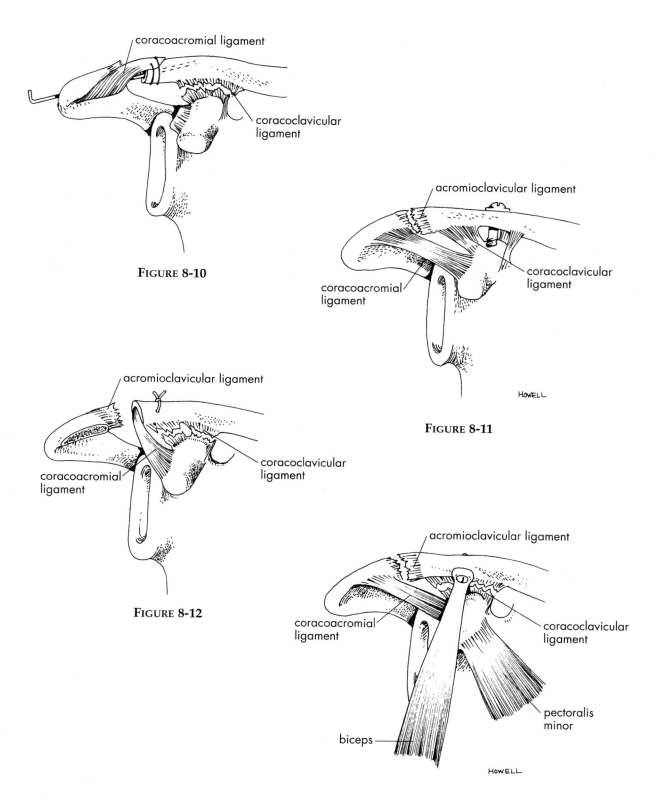

Figure 8-10

Figure 8-11

Figure 8-12

Figure 8-13

SURGICAL TECHNIQUE

Positioning

The patient may be placed in the "beach chair" position (see Fig. 2-1). It is advantageous to have a headrest or to use a semi-sitting position (see Fig. 2-2) to allow an approach to the superior aspect of the shoulder. The arm is draped free following prepping in the usual fashion. The drapes are carried high onto the neck to allow access to the superior aspect of the shoulder.

Approach

A 3-in. S-shaped incision is made from the acromioclavicular joint beginning 1 cm posterior to the joint, then brought inferiorly toward the coracoid process, curving gently medially and then distally (Fig. 8-14). The skin incision may be altered to fit surgeon preference. The aponeurosis of the deltoid and the trapezius as it inserts on the superior aspect of the clavicle are incised over the distal 2 to 3 cm of the clavicle. The deltoid is incised off the anterior clavicle from the coracoid to the acromioclavicular joint (Fig. 8-15). As this flap of deltoid is elevated, the tip of the coracoid process will be palpated and may be visualized. This flap of deltoid is tagged, capturing both the superior and the inferior fascial planes. For reconstruction of chronic separations, a distal clavicle resection is performed (see distal clavicle excision, p. 240).

Procedure

The initial step might be to place sutures in the stumps of the torn coracoclavicular ligaments (Fig. 8-16). A small elevator is used to subperiosteally dissect about the neck of the coracoid. Extreme caution is exercised during this portion of the procedure because of the proximity of neurovascular structures lying inferiorly and medially to the coracoid. A blunt, curved instrument is used to complete the dissection from lateral to medial beneath the neck of the coracoid. The surgeon's index finger is placed along the medial border of the coracoid to palpate the instrument as it comes through the inferior surface. Ideally, this instrument should be passed immediately posterior to the insertion of the coracoacromial ligament onto the coracoid, thus preserving the attachment of the ligament as well as placing the suture as close to the base of the coracoid as possible. This will prevent later migration of the graft material and loosening of the repair.

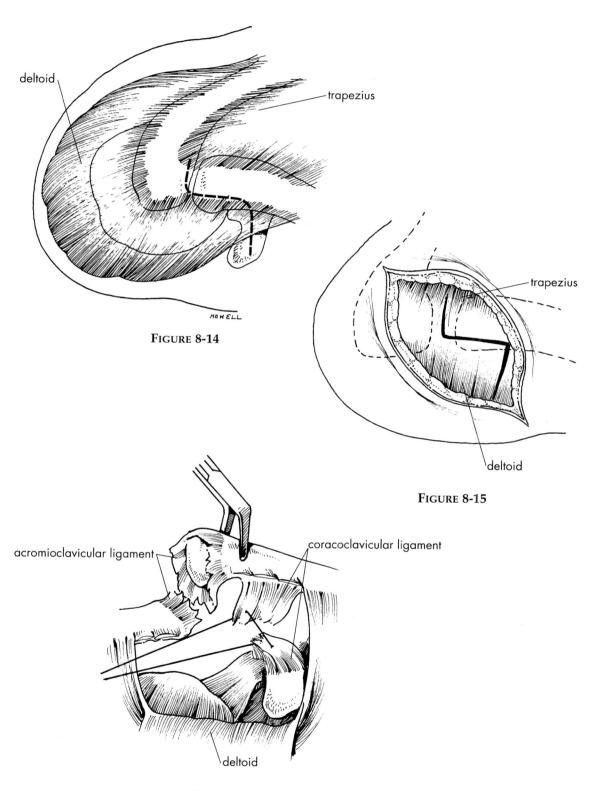

deltoid

trapezius

HOWELL

FIGURE 8-14

trapezius

deltoid

FIGURE 8-15

acromioclavicular ligament

coracoclavicular ligament

deltoid

FIGURE 8-16

When the surgeon is comfortable that a passageway has been created along the undersurface of the coracoid, a suture passer from the Rowe-Bankart tray is loaded with a No. 1 Surgilon and gently placed about the inferior surface of the coracoid. Fig. 8-17 shows the suture passer coursing posterior to the coracoacromial ligament near the base of the coracoid and exiting on the medial aspect. Fig. 8-18 shows an anterior view of this step. One end of this suture is then pulled through and tied to the graft of braided PDS. The graft is then passed in a retrograde fashion under the coracoid. A 3/16-in. drill hole is made as far laterally as is practical on the clavicle, and the graft material is passed back through this hole. A Bristow elevator is then positioned on the superior aspect of the clavicle, pushing it inferiorly into a reduced position (Fig. 8-19). The graft is tied and the stumps of the ruptured coracoclavicular ligaments are repaired with multiple stitches of a No. 1 nonabsorbable suture material (Fig. 8-16). It is important when placing the graft from the coracoid to the clavicle that the material be placed through a drill hole that is anterior in the clavicle (Fig. 8-20). If the graft is placed around the clavicle, or if the drill hole is posterior, the joint is malreduced with anterior displacement of the outer clavicle (Fig. 8-21).

It is preferred, even in acute situations, to provide additional backup to this reconstruction with a coracoacromial ligament transfer (a modified Weaver-Dunn) procedure. This procedure involves a release of the acromial attachment of the coracoacromial ligament with a small wafer of bone. In acute situations, the ligament is passed through a drill hole and sutured onto itself (Fig. 8-22).

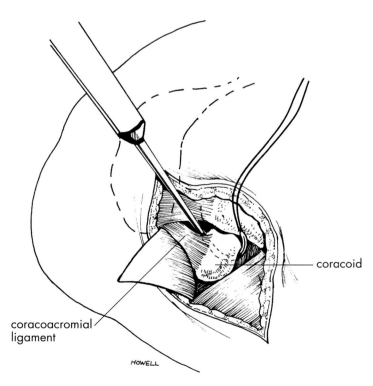

coracoid

coracoacromial ligament

HOWELL

FIGURE 8-17

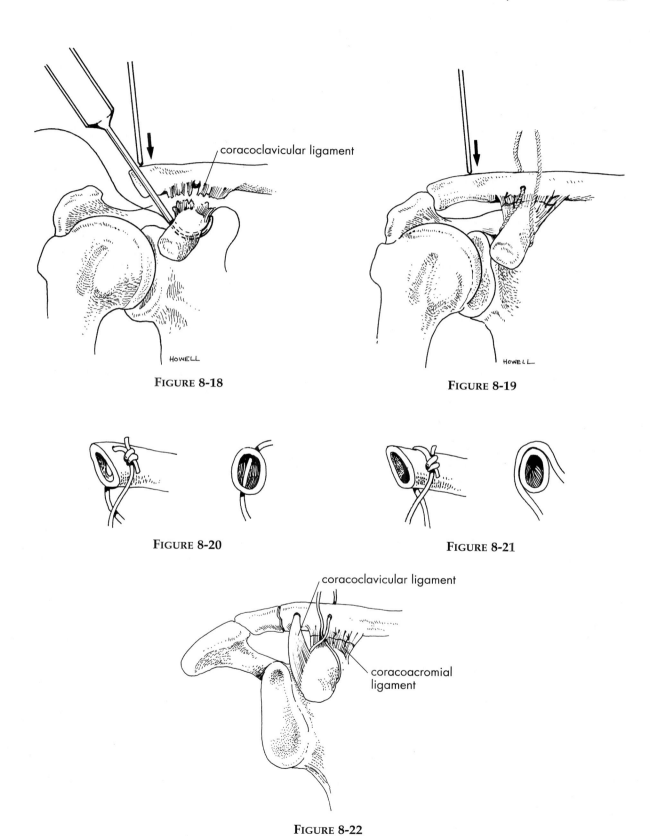

coracoclavicular ligament

HOWELL

FIGURE 8-18

HOWELL

FIGURE 8-19

FIGURE 8-20

FIGURE 8-21

coracoclavicular ligament

coracoacromial
ligament

FIGURE 8-22

In a chronic situation, the ligament is transferred to the intramedullary canal of the distal clavicle and sutures are placed through a drill hole in the superior aspect of the clavicle lateral to the previous reconstruction (Fig. 8-23). A small piece of bone can be excised from the acromion with the ligament and pulled into the medullary canal of the outer clavicle. This step will provide additional stability to the repair and provide autogenous backup once the PDS suture graft loses its strength. Hewson suture passers are helpful in passage of the sutures through the canal and the drill hole. If fixation in either an acute or chronic situation is inadequate, autogenous palmaris longus tendon graft may be added to the construct by passing it under the coracoid and through the same drill holes as the PDS suture.

Closure

The deltotrapezial fascia is repaired in an imbricated fashion on the superior surface of the clavicle to further reinforce the repair (Fig. 8-24). Subcutaneous tissue and skin are closed in layers with a running subcuticular stitch. The patient is placed into a light compressive dressing and sling immobilization. A drain is optional, but seldom necessary.

POSTOPERATIVE CARE (SEE CHAPTER 11)

Because of the significant forces applied to this reconstruction, the patient is kept in sling immobilization for the first 3 weeks. The patient is allowed to remove the sling for showering and for gentle pendulum exercises, but formal range of motion exercises are delayed until approximately 3 weeks. At that point, gentle active and passive motion below horizontal is begun. All motions are kept below 90° of forward elevation for at least 6 weeks to avoid additional stresses to the repair. At 6 weeks, motion is increased and gentle resistive exercises are started. At 2 months, isokinetic strengthening may be started. Heavy manual labor and athletic endeavors are avoided for at least 3 months.

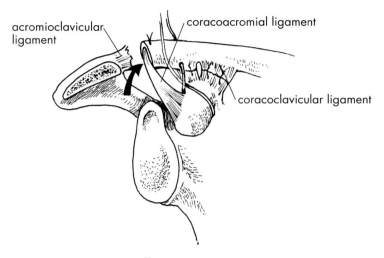

FIGURE 8-23

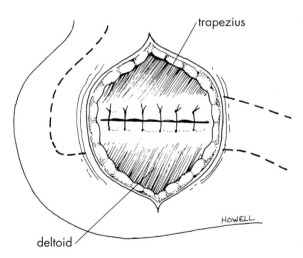

FIGURE 8-24

Coracoclavicular Screw Fixation in Acute and Chronic Acromioclavicular Separations

GENERAL CONSIDERATIONS

In both acute and chronic situations of clavicular separations, screw fixation is a reasonable option. In the acute setting, this technique allows stabilization of the clavicle, during which time the coracoclavicular ligaments, which are repaired at the time of the operative procedure, are allowed to heal. Screw fixation is a temporary form of stabilization. Some surgeons remove the screw in 6 weeks, although this is not mandatory. If used in an acute situation, screw stabilization with concomitant ligament repair is usually adequate. If the separation is chronic, coracoclavicular ligament reconstruction is often impossible and the repair should be backed up with a coracoacromial ligament transfer, as described in the previous section. In the chronic setting, the outer clavicle is excised (see outer clavicle excision, p. 240).

Indications

This type of repair may be used in acute or chronic Grade III separations in healthy, active individuals. Relative indications would be a Grade III separation in a throwing athlete or a patient who does heavy manual labor.

Expectations

The expectations are similar to those for the previous reconstruction. The majority of these individuals, especially in acute situations, will achieve a very stable, cosmetically pleasing acromioclavicular joint. In chronic separations the repair will eliminate a good deal of the symptoms of fatigue that these individuals note after their separation. Return to normal work and athletics can begin at 3 months.

SURGICAL TECHNIQUE
Positioning

The "beach chair" position (see Fig. 2-1) is used with padding beneath the involved scapula to elevate the shoulder more than in the standard "beach chair" position. The semi-sitting position may also be used (see Fig. 2-2). If films are to be taken intraoperatively, it is advantageous to place a film under the patient at this time. Drapes should be placed high on the neck, and a headrest is helpful.

Approach

A 3-in. S-shaped incision is made from the acromioclavicular joint beginning 1 cm posterior to the joint, then brought inferiorly toward the coracoid process, curving gently medially and then distally (see Fig. 8-14). The deltoid is released from the anterior aspect of the clavicle and is split bluntly along the orientation of its fibers (see Fig. 8-15). This step provides visualization of the disrupted acromioclavicular joint and the coracoclavicular ligaments on the undersurface of the clavicle (see Fig. 8-16).

Procedure

The acromioclavicular joint is exposed and debrided. Any retained meniscal fragments are excised. Any chondral damage is appropriately addressed. The coracoclavicular ligaments are identified, and tag sutures are placed, anticipating a subsequent repair (see Fig. 8-16). To achieve this, we use a No. 2 nonabsorbable braided suture in a figure eight fashion. The superior surface of the coracoid is palpated, and any interposed soft tissue is gently freed. The clavicle is then grasped with a towel clip and held in a reduced position.

With the clavicle reduced, a drill hole is made through both cortices of the clavicle, aiming directly to the base of the coracoid (Fig. 8-25). The drill diameter for the clavicle and the coracoid is based on screw selection. This diameter may be ensured either by direct visualization or by palpation of the base of the coracoid before drilling. As described by Rockwood, it is important that both cortices of the base of the coracoid are incorporated into the fixation. Thus, the drill bit must be directed in a vertical fashion to pass through both of these cortices, yet avoiding injury to neurovascular structures deep to the coracoid (Fig. 8-25).

While continuing to hold the clavicle in a reduced position, the appropriate length cancellous screw (or Bosworth, Rockwood, or AO screw) is applied and tightened to ensure appropriate position of the clavicle relative to the acromial facet. It is important not to overtighten the screw, but merely reapproximate the articular surfaces (Fig. 8-26). The final step is to tie the previously placed sutures in the coracoclavicular ligaments (Fig. 8-27). In chronic cases, the outer clavicle is excised and the coracoacromial ligament may be transferred (Weaver-Dunn procedure) to the exposed intramedullary canal of the clavicle (Fig. 8-23).

Closure

The deltoid is allowed to fall back into its normal position and then repaired to the trapezial fascia superiorly, using a nonabsorbable suture material (Fig. 8-24). Subcutaneous tissue and skin are closed in a standard fashion, and the patient is placed in a shoulder immobilizer.

POSTOPERATIVE CARE (SEE CHAPTER 11)

The postoperative care closely follows that of the previous procedure with a sling for the first 3 weeks and then gentle pendulum exercises. The patient is not allowed to perform any significant degree of active or passive motion. At 3 weeks the patient is started on range of motion exercises, slowly regaining forward elevation. At 5 to 6 weeks, forward elevation beyond 90° is encouraged and gentle resisted exercises may be started. Isokinetic strengthening may be initiated at 8 weeks with an anticipated resumption of athletic and work-related activities at 3 months.

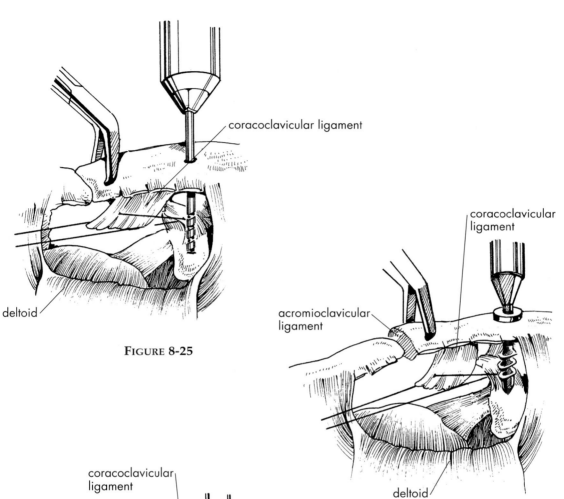

FIGURE 8-25

FIGURE 8-26

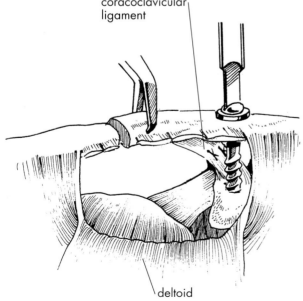

FIGURE 8-27

Acromioclavicular Pinning in Acute Acromioclavicular Separations
GENERAL CONSIDERATIONS

In acute separations, an option is pinning of the joint preceded by a limited arthrotomy. This option allows visualization of the joint for debridement and accurate reduction before pinning. Many devices are available for this technique, including smooth and threaded K-wires, Knowles' pins, and Simmons' pins. All of these devices provide temporary fixation of the joint while the reapposed coracoclavicular ligaments heal. Their disadvantage is the violation of the joint surface and the fact that the ligaments, although theoretically reapposed, are not anatomically repaired. In addition, a second procedure is required to remove the fixation.

Indications

This technique may be applied to acute Grade IV or greater separations in healthy, active individuals. Individuals with a Grade III injury who participate in significant overhead throwing or manual labor may also be considered.

Expectations

Expectations with this procedure would suggest that one could obtain restoration of normal shoulder appearance and anticipate return to athletic and work-related endeavors at approximately 3 to 4 months.

SURGICAL TECHNIQUE
Positioning

The patient may be placed in the "beach chair" position (see Fig. 2-1). A headrest or the semi-sitting position is also helpful (see Fig. 2-2). The drapes must be placed high on the neck to allow a superior approach to the shoulder. The patient is brought into a very lateral position on the table with the arm draped free. The head is turned to the contralateral side. Before the procedure begins, the fluoroscope should be brought into the room and a trial reduction of the joint performed with imaging in both the anteroposterior and the axillary planes. This is especially important if a percutaneous closed pinning of the joint is to be performed. If an open reduction is planned, placement of the pins across the joint will be verified under direct vision.

Approach

In open pinnings, the acromioclavicular joint is visualized, using a 3 cm oblique incision made directly over the joint (see Figs. 2-36 and 2-37). This incision is taken down through the subcutaneous tissue with hemostasis secured by electrocautery. The deltotrapezial aponeurosis is visualized and is incised transversely along the line of the middle of the clavicle. Subperiosteally, the joint is exposed (see Fig. 8-5, A).

Procedure

The articular surfaces of the distal clavicle and acromion are inspected. Retractors are placed under the distal clavicle (Fig. 8-28). All interposed soft tissue and meniscal fragments are removed, and the joint is reduced. The pinning of the joint may be done in either an antegrade or a retrograde fashion. If the acromial facet is readily visualized, a pin may be placed from the joint to the lateral aspect of the acromion and through the skin. If a Knowles' screw or Simmons' pin is to be used, both threaded devices, a small incision is made on the lateral aspect of the acromion, and the screws are brought from the lateral acromion back medially across the joint into the clavicle (Fig. 8-29). The advantage of this technique is that it allows excellent visualization of the joint, debridement of any damaged tissue and/or chondral tissue, and anatomical reduction of the joint.

If a percutaneous technique is to be used, a small incision only to allow introduction of the fixation device is made at the lateral margin of the acromion. A small rongeur bite of the lateral acromion will allow one to start the fixation device. The joint itself is not exposed. With this technique, the clavicle is held in a reduced position and the wire is directed across the joint, using image amplification principally in the AP plane. Pin position in the anteroposterior direction may be confirmed, using the axillary view initially and then converting back to the AP view for advancing the pin across the joint. Several different devices may be used for this fixation: smooth K-wires, Knowles' pins, Simmons' pins, or cannulated screws. The larger the device, the greater the risk of damage to the articular surface. One must weigh the risk of such joint injury against the strength of the fixation device. However, historically, devices placed across this joint have not proven to lead to a greater incidence of degenerative disease.

Closure

In the case of the open arthrotomy, the fascial layers are reapproximated with a nonabsorbable suture and the subcutaneous tissue and skin are closed appropriately. The patient is placed into a sling immobilizer. If the joint has been pinned percutaneously, the pin may be left out through the skin or, if adequate soft tissue is present, it may be buried just beneath it for later removal. If the pins are left protruding through the skin, office removal is feasible.

POSTOPERATIVE CARE (SEE CHAPTER 11)
Open Reduction

The rehabilitation following open reduction and internal fixation requires a temporary period of immobilization of approximately 3 weeks followed by passive and active range of motion with resisted exercises beginning at approximately 6 weeks. The fixation device is removed at 6 to 8 weeks.

Percutaneous Pinning

Immobilization is carried out for approximately 3 weeks, and then gentle range of motion exercises are performed and the pins removed at approximately 6 weeks. Active exercises begin at 6 weeks, and resisted exercises are added at 8 to 10 weeks.

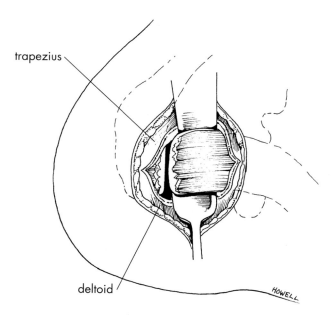

trapezius

deltoid

FIGURE 8-28

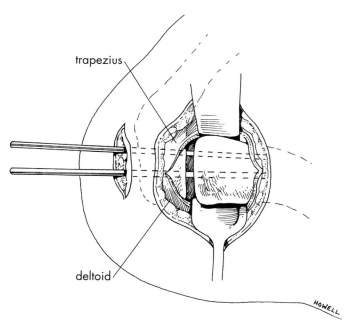

trapezius

deltoid

FIGURE 8-29

Sternoclavicular Joint

9

Introduction

Surgery for the sternoclavicular joint is rarely indicated. The pathology seen in the sternoclavicular joint consists of fractures, arthritis, fixed anterior dislocation, posterior dislocation, and an unstable sternoclavicular joint.

The concern regarding sternoclavicular surgery is related to the neurovascular structures that lie just posterior to the inner end of the clavicle. A related concern that may be unappreciated involves the marked depth posteriorly that the inner end of the clavicle occupies. Finally, operations on the inner clavicle seem to carry a lower success rate with a higher morbidity rate than many operations about the shoulder.

Resection of Medial Clavicle

GENERAL CONSIDERATIONS

Indications

The indications for resecting the medial end of the clavicle relate to destructive changes of the sternoclavicular joint with disabling pain and an obvious failure of a conservative program. It is rarely indicated and should be avoided if possible.

Expectations

The expectations regarding resection of the inner clavicle are somewhat guarded. Not all patients obtain pain relief. If pain relief is obtained, however, good functional return should follow.

SURGICAL TECHNIQUE

Positioning

The patient is placed in the "beach chair" position (see Fig. 2-1). The inner end of the clavicle can be either square draped or the entire extremity draped free. The inner clavicle and the sternum are outlined with a marking pencil. The semi-sitting position may be used (see Fig. 2-2).

Approach

A 3-cm skin incision may be transverse, centered over the sternoclavicular joint, or extended along the clavicle (Fig. 9-1). The subcutaneous tissue is reflected, and the underlying periosteum is identified.

Procedure

The periosteum is incised, staying in the mid portion of the inner end of the clavicle, and carefully stripped off with a sharp instrument superiorly and inferiorly. The ligaments at the sternoclavicular joint are incised at right angles to identify the joint. Caution should be exercised during dissection to avoid damage to the vital structures just posterior to the inner end of the clavicle. Some form of retractor, such as a Lane, can be positioned carefully. One retractor should be placed superiorly and one inferiorly to lever the inner end of the clavicle forward as much as possible (Fig. 9-2). An osteotomy cut can be carefully performed, either with an osteotome or a power saw, excising approximately 2 cm from the inner end of the clavicle (Fig. 9-3). It may be safer to pass a Gigli saw carefully around the clavicle and cut it forward. A towel clip can then be placed on the inner end of the clavicle, which can be carefully dissected free of the posterior soft tissue attachments (Fig. 9-4). Note at this point the suprisingly posterior extension of the proximal clavicle (Fig. 9-5).

Closure

The dead space must be carefully closed, and the subcutaneous tissue and the skin are closed in the usual fashion over a drain.

POSTOPERATIVE CARE (SEE CHAPTER 11)

A firm pressure dressing will minimize bleeding. Gentle range of motion exercises can rapidly progress through Phases I, II and III, as pain permits. Passive Phase I can be started the day of surgery and continued for 5 to 7 days. Phase II active exercises can begin at approximately 1 week. Resisted exercises should be delayed until 3 months.

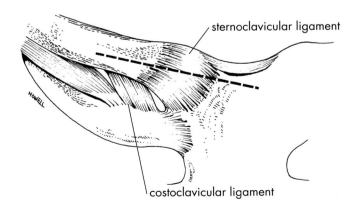

FIGURE 9-1

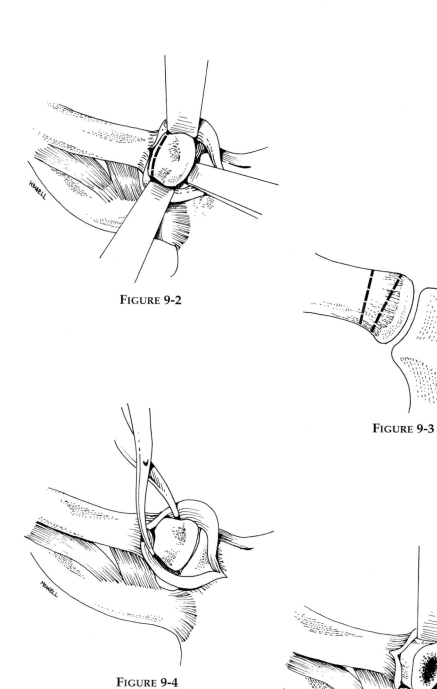

FIGURE 9-2

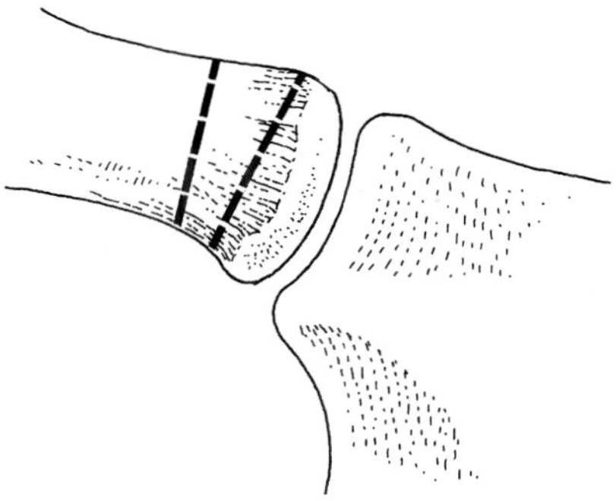

FIGURE 9-3

FIGURE 9-4

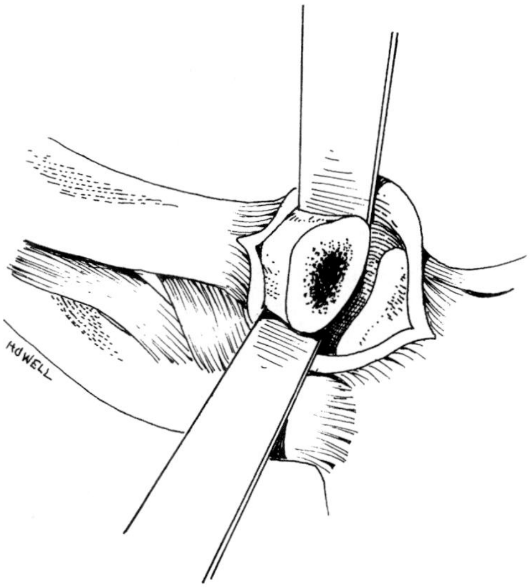

FIGURE 9-5

Posterior Dislocation
GENERAL CONSIDERATIONS

An acute posterior dislocation of the inner end of the clavicle is not only significantly painful but can cause vascular or respiratory compromise. It can represent a medical emergency requiring immediate reduction, often with immediate transfer to an operating room for a general anesthetic.

SURGICAL TECHNIQUE
Positioning

The patient is positioned supine on the operating table. Under general anesthesia, an inflatable cuff or roll can be placed in the midline between the scapulae to thrust the chest forward. Extension traction of the abducted arm might achieve reduction. If this maneuver does not work, the inner clavicle area can be prepped, and a towel clip can be inserted around the inner end of the clavicle through the skin, pulling the clavicle forward to a reduced position (Fig. 9-6). Failure to achieve reduction with a towel clip may require an open reduction. The inner clavicle is then prepped and draped in the usual fashion. The arm should be free so that it can be manipulated.

Approach

A transverse incision is made over the inner end of the clavicle, for a distance of approximately 3 cm (Fig. 9-1).

Procedure

The defect is identified, and the soft tissues around the inner end of the clavicle are carefully dissected free. With a towel clip or grasping instrument placed around the inner end, and under direct visualization, the inner clavicle is manipulated into a reduced position (Fig. 9-4). Following reduction, stability should be assessed and the best arm position determined for postoperative stability. Usually following open or closed reduction, stability is secure, although certain positions may allow subtle resubluxations.

Closure

Following open reduction, subcutaneous tissue and skin are closed in the usual fashion, and the arm is appropriately positioned in a stable situation for short-term immobilization. A drain is unnecessary.

POSTOPERATIVE CARE (SEE CHAPTER 11)

The arm should be kept in a sling for approximately 2 to 3 weeks, followed by gentle range of motion exercises progressing rapidly from Phase I to Phase III.

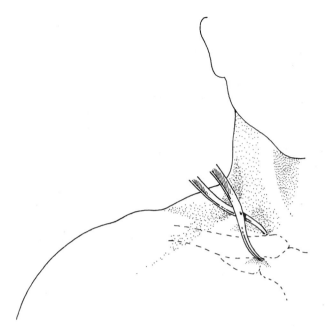

FIGURE 9-6

Reconstruction for Sternoclavicular Instability
GENERAL CONSIDERATIONS
The sternoclavicular joint may become unstable, particularly in the ligamentous-lax individual. It may occur following a traumatic insult, or its onset may be spontaneous. Surgical reconstruction is rare because most patients are not symptomatic enough and the surgery is very challenging.

Indications
In the very painful and unstable situation that is resistant to conservative measures, occasionally reconstruction may be attempted.

Contraindication
The contraindications to such a procedure may be in psychologically disturbed people.

Expectations
The expectations regarding surgical reconstruction are guarded. The successful outcome of such a procedure is a return to a relatively normal functioning shoulder.

SURGICAL TECHNIQUE
Positioning
The patient is placed in the "beach chair" position (see Fig. 2-1). The clavicle can be square draped, although it is probably more appropriate to drape the arm free in case manipulation is required. The semi-sitting position is another option (see Fig. 2-2).

Approach
A transverse incision, approximately 3 to 5 cm long, is centered over the inner end of the clavicle (see Fig. 9-1).

Procedure
The periosteal layer of the inner end of the clavicle is identified and carefully stripped (see Fig. 9-2). The inner 1 cm of the clavicle is excised as previously described (see Fig. 9-5). Dissection is taken down to the first rib just below the inner aspect of the clavicle, approximately 2 to 3 cm from the sternoclavicular joint. The first rib must be carefully identified, and the periosteum must be incised in the direction of the rib and carefully stripped off superiorly and inferiorly. A passageway is created very carefully behind the first rib. Careful subperiosteal dissection is performed, being careful not to penetrate the pleural cavity. The subclavius muscle, which lies inferior to the clavicle, is identified and dissected, leaving it attached medially so that it can be used as autogenous tissue in the reconstruction. The subclavius, however, is often not strong autogenous tissue. A better option is to add an autogenous palmaris longus graft. It is advisable to add some form of synthetic material along with the subclavius, passing it around the first rib and through drill holes in the clavicle placed at its inner end. We have been using several strands of braided PDS suture. These can be tied in a figure eight fashion. Fig. 9-7 shows a method of passing some form of synthetic suture around the first rib and through the inner clavicle. Fig. 9-8 shows subclavius and synthetic sutures. Fig. 9-9 shows the palmaris longus graft.

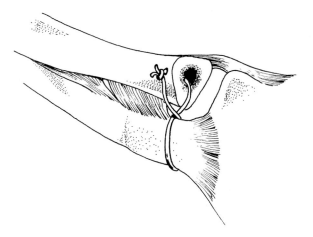

FIGURE 9-7

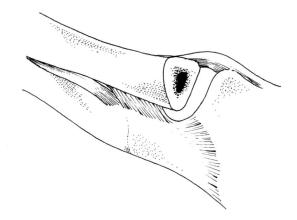

FIGURE 9-8

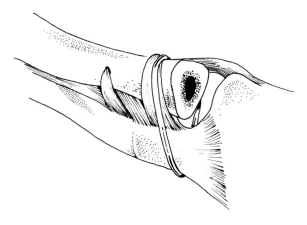

FIGURE 9-9

Closure

After completion of the procedure, the subcutaneous tissue and skin are closed in the usual fashion. A drain is usually not required. The surgeon must be alert to the possibility of a pneumothorax and an immediate postoperative chest x-ray is advisable. During the procedure, submersing the wound in water would demonstrate any leakage of air from the lungs. The surgeon should make preoperative preparations for a thoracostomy tube in case a pneumothorax occurs.

POSTOPERATIVE CARE (SEE CHAPTER 11)

Postoperative care consists of temporary immobilization and the use of a sling for approximately 3 to 4 weeks, followed by gentle range of motion. The patient can progress rapidly through the phases of rehabilitation as pain permits. Phase I starts at 4 weeks, lasting for 2 weeks; Phase II begins at 6 weeks; and Phase III begins at 10 weeks.

Arthroscopy

10

Introduction

During the past decade, arthroscopy of the shoulder has moved from an experimental, seldom-used procedure to the forefront of the subspecialty of shoulder surgery. Its use has greatly enhanced our diagnostic capabilities and has helped with an understanding of disease processes of the shoulder. With surgical applications in acromioplasty, stabilization of the glenohumeral joint, arthroplasty of the acromioclavicular joint, rotator cuff repairs, and chondroplasties, its therapeutic effects are being explored and realized. Although many techniques used on the knee are applicable, the glenohumeral and acromioclavicular articulations represent a distinct group of joints with their own set of problems.

Portal placement is extremely important and, in many instances, the learning curve can be steeper and longer than in the knee. If a pump is used, a system that senses pressure only at the terminal part of the arthroscope is advantageous. This type of system lessens distension and extravasation problems, such as swelling. An inflow augmented by a pump system that senses through a separate portal may result in significant extracapsular fluid extravasation. The surgeon must be cautious in such instances to avoid potential neurovascular compromise. As our interest in glenohumeral stabilization has increased, the need for arm suspension units and traction has grown. With such traction, a new group of potential associated complications, such as neurological compromise, exists. The surgeon interested in shoulder arthroscopy must be mindful of such potential problems.

Basic Set-Up

Successful arthroscopy requires the union of a well-trained staff, adequate anesthesia, appropriate instrumentation, and an experienced surgeon. Inherent in this procedure is an efficient and organized operating room set-up. Using the lateral decubitus position, the arm may be suspended with a traction device from the foot of the table (see Fig. 2-5). Traction can safely be provided with 3-liter IV bags, which are approximately 10 lbs each. The arm on the down side of the patient is brought out into slight forward elevation with an axillary roll to prevent neurovascular compromise. The anesthesiologist is at the head of the table and the scrub nurse may pass instruments from either side of the table, more commonly from the side opposite the surgeon. In cases of arthroscopic acromioplasties, one monitor across from the surgeon is adequate. In stabilizations, it may be necessary to have a monitor on both sides of the patient with the surgeon standing at the head, working from both posterior and anterior.

If the sitting position is to be used, a specific table that not only stabilizes the head (that is, a headrest), but also allows exposure to the involved shoulder, is helpful (see Fig. 2-2). The type of anesthetic used will depend on several factors, including the patient's health, age, size, and type of procedure. Scalene blocks are ideal in the outpatient ambulatory setting. They provide perioperative and postoperative pain relief, allow early patient discharge, and avoid the risks of a general anesthetic. They do require a skilled anesthesiologist and a cooperative patient. The sitting position is best with an interscalene block since the patient is able to control head position. General anesthesia in the sitting position is somewhat awkward because of difficulty in controlling the head.

In the lateral decubitus position during routine diagnostic procedures, assessment of rotator cuff lesions, or both, the arm is suspended at 30° to 40° of abduction with 10 lbs of traction (see Fig. 2-5). The arm is then flexed forward 15°, and the body is rolled back 20° to 30° posterior to the vertical plane (see Fig. 2-6). This places the glenoid parallel with the floor. This position allows ease of visualization of the anterior glenoid structures, especially during stabilizations. The amount of arm abduction and flexion varies according to the specific procedure. Diagnostic procedures are best accomplished with 45° of abduction to allow distraction of the humeral head. Subacromial work (that is, decompressions) requires less abduction (approximately 10° to 20°) to bring the greater tuberosity down away from the acromion. Instability procedures often require a second traction sling about the upper arm, directed cephalad, pulling the head laterally away from the glenoid (see Figs. 2-7 and 2-8). This exposes the anterior glenolabral complex and inferior glenohumeral ligament, which facilitates instrumentation of these structures, allowing repair of a Bankart lesion.

PORTALS

Proper portal placement in shoulder arthroscopy is crucial to ensure adequate visualization and ease of surgical techniques. Because of the many soft tissue planes, it is important that the surgeon avoid extracapsular fluid inflow. This inflow will result in a diminished intraarticular space, poor visualization, and difficulty with the procedure. Portals should be made and maintained with strict adherence to external topography and internal anatomy. The basic portals, their positions, and uses are as follows:

Posterior Portal (Fig. 10-1)
  Position: 2 cm inferior to the posterolateral corner of the acromion.
  Uses: Standard viewing portal for diagnostic arthroscopy of the glenohumeral joint and for acromioplasty.

Direct Posterior Portal (Fig. 10-2)
  Position: 1 cm inferior to the posterior acromion in the middle of the posterior acromion.
  Uses: Advantageous portal for arthroscopic subacromial decompression allowing visualization of the anteromedial and anterolateral corners.

Lateral Portal (Fig. 10-3)
  Position: 1 to 2 cm posterior, 2 to 3 cm lateral to the anterolateral corner of the acromion. This portal should be anterior to a line drawn from the posterior margin of the acromioclavicular joint and perpendicular to the lateral margin of the acromion.

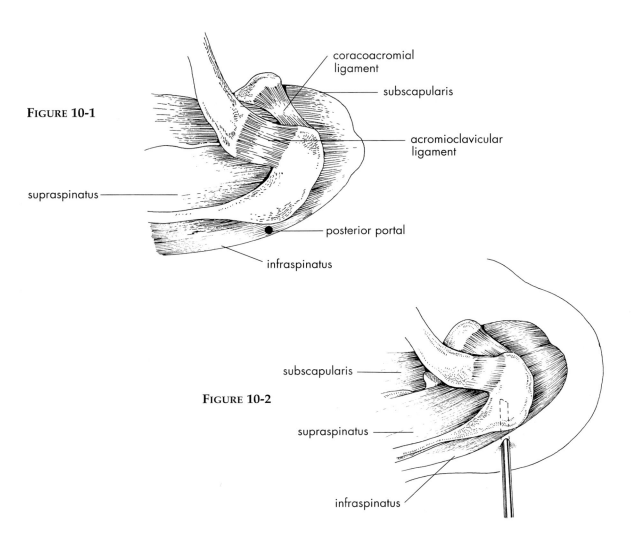

FIGURE 10-1

coracoacromial ligament

subscapularis

acromioclavicular ligament

supraspinatus

posterior portal

infraspinatus

FIGURE 10-2

subscapularis

supraspinatus

infraspinatus

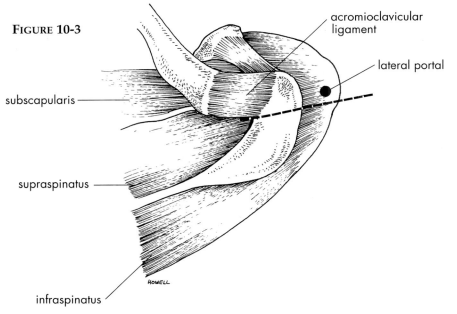

FIGURE 10-3

acromioclavicular ligament

lateral portal

subscapularis

supraspinatus

infraspinatus

HOWELL

Uses: Working portal for instrumentation during arthroscopic acromio-plasties. This portal may be used for visualization during acromioplasty with instrumentation coming from the posterior. This portal is also used as a viewing portal for resections of the distal clavicle.

Anterior Portal (Fig. 10-4)
Position: 1 cm lateral and 1 cm superior to the coracoid process. This portal is often established from inside out, using switching sticks to ensure proper positioning.
Uses: Ideal portal for inflow, instrumentation, or both during arthroscopic stabilizations, labral resections, synovectomies, and chondroplasties.

Anterosuperior Portal (Fig. 10-5)
Position: 1 cm inferior and 1 cm lateral to the acromioclavicular joint.
Uses: Visualization portal for anterior reconstructions and for some acromioclavicular joint instrumentation.

Superior Portal - "Neviaser Portal" (Fig. 10-6)
Position: 1 cm medial to the "soft spot" posterior to the acromioclavicular joint. The cannula is directed in a lateral and posterior direction.
Uses: Best used for inflow. This portal may also be used as a superior portal for arthroscopic synovectomies.

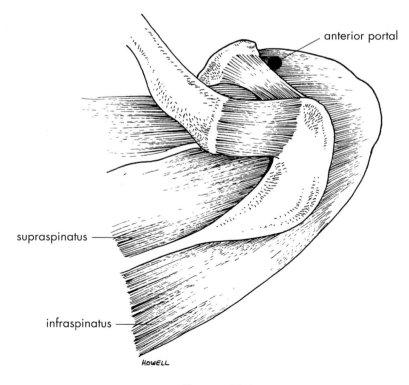

FIGURE 10-4

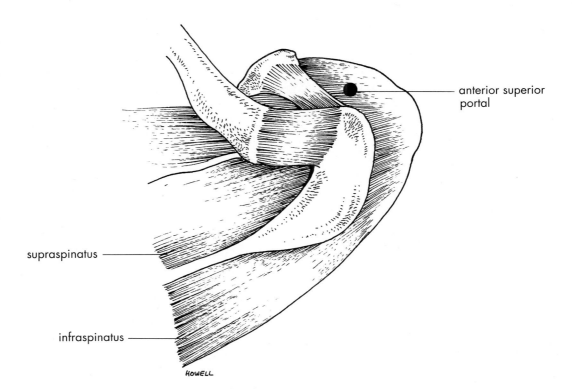

anterior superior
portal

supraspinatus

infraspinatus

HOWELL

FIGURE 10-5

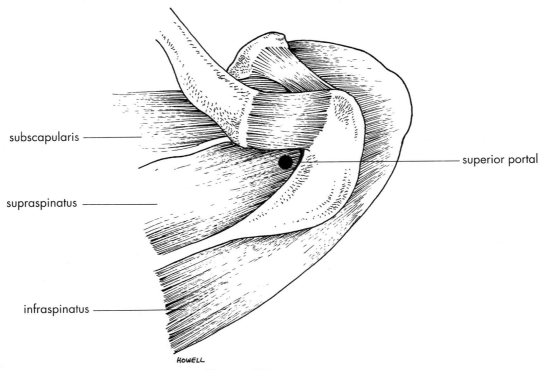

subscapularis

superior portal

supraspinatus

infraspinatus

HOWELL

FIGURE 10-6

Arthroscopic Subacromial Decompression (ASD)

GENERAL CONSIDERATIONS

Arthroscopic subacromial decompression (ASD) for chronic impingement tendinitis has become a viable treatment option for impingement tendinitis of the shoulder. First described and popularized by Dr. Ellman, this procedure demands a high level of arthroscopic skill on the part of the surgeon. Not only does the technique allow for decompression of the subacromial space, but it also provides an opportunity for intraarticular glenohumeral inspection, thus minimizing the chances for errors in diagnosis.

Indications

ASD is indicated in patients with pain from chronic impingement tendinitis failing an adequate trial of conservative management (6 months). The presence of any underlying instability must be considered because a decompression alone may fail. Acromioclavicular joint pathology and cuff tears should also be defined preoperatively and may, in some cases, be addressed at the time of ASD.

Expectations

Relief of pain and return to functional use of the shoulder for most activities occur in 75% to 85% of patients in most published reports. Although postoperative morbidity is less, return to work and restoration of motion may take as long as with the standard open acromioplasty. Symptoms usually resolve between 2 and 3 months, with return to sports and labor activities at approximately 3 to 4 months if this goal is to be achieved.

SURGICAL TECHNIQUE
Positioning

The procedure may be performed in either the lateral decubitus (see Fig. 2-4) or semi-sitting position (see Fig. 2-2). Our preference is the regular "beach chair" position (see Fig. 2-1). In the lateral decubitus position, a bean bag is used to stabilize the body. An axillary roll is placed beneath the down side axilla to protect the brachial plexus. The arm is suspended in a slight degree of abduction, approximately 20°, with 10 lbs of traction, using an IV bag. Elbows, knees, and heels are protected. It is important to outline the acromion, acromioclavicular joints, and other bony landmarks before proceeding. A line parallel with the posterior border of the clavicle perpendicular to the lateral edge of the acromion indicates the posterior extent of the planned acromioplasty (Fig. 10-3).

Procedure

As in all arthroscopic shoulder procedures, the glenohumeral joint is initially inspected from a posterior portal. The joint may be entered by one of two techniques, the first being that of needle insufflation with 30 to 50 cc of saline, thus making cannula introduction somewhat easier. The difficulty with this technique occurs when the sharp needle point engages the head or scapular neck, making joint penetration difficult.

The second technique is by direct cannula introduction with a blunt trochar. In both instances, the glenohumeral joint is palpated and the trochar is directed toward the coracoid process. The blunt trochar is always used to enter the joint, thereby minimizing the risk of chondral injury, which is possible with a sharp trochar. Upon first visualization in the joint, the view will be white. Syringe insufflation allows determination of whether the joint has been entered before the pump is started. Diagnostic arthroscopy is then carried out by the posterior portal. If no surgery is required within the joint, a 14-gauge needle can be inserted in the anterosuperior portal to establish flow for better visualization. If intraarticular surgery is necessary for rotator cuff debridement, labral debridement, or removal of loose bodies, an anterior portal is used for inflow, introduction of instrumentation, such as a shaver system, or both.

Upon completion of the intraarticular portion of the case, the anterior instrumentation is removed and the arthroscope is redirected, sometimes using the same posterior portal, into the subacromial space. Our preference is to use a direct posterior portal for the camera, which facilitates better visualization of the anterior corners (see Fig. 10-2). Introduction of the cannula into the subacromial space is achieved by backing the cannula out of the posterior capsule and then redirecting it 20° to 30° cephalad until the undersurface of the acromion is palpated. This is an ideal time to use the blunt trochar to free subacromial adhesions and to create a larger subacromial space within which to perform the decompression. The trochar may be used to define the contour and thickness of the coracoacromial ligament and the anterolateral and anteromedial margins of the undersurface of the acromion. If a separate portal is necessary for inflow, it may be established using either the anterosuperior portal (see Fig. 10-5) or one of the two posterior portals (see Figs. 10-1, 10-2 and 10-9). An inflow pressure system is best and avoids the need for an additional portal for inflow. The outflow is through the operating instruments, which are brought in through the lateral portal. The surgeon may find, after beginning the debridement of the subacromial space, that the standard posterior portal is inadequate for visualization and may need to switch to the posterolateral portal for viewing (see Fig. 10-10). This is especially true in cases with a profound hook to the acromion where the anterior resection must be anterior to the midsubstance of the acromion.

Needle localizations may be used as markers for the anterolateral and anteromedial corners of the acromion (Figs. 10-7 and 10-8). These markers are placed by palpation and assist with the intraarticular visualization of the margins of the acromion so that an adequate decompression is ensured. This technique is shown in Fig. 10-7, looking from above, and Fig. 10-8, looking from posterior to anterior. These figures show the position of the needles relative to the anterolateral and medial corners of the acromion.

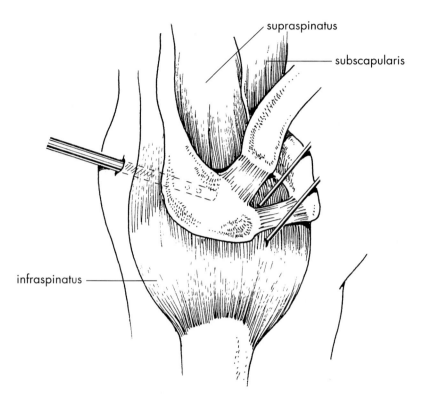

FIGURE 10-7

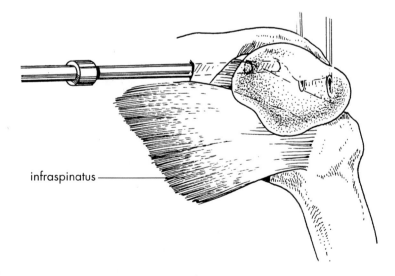

FIGURE 10-8

Fig. 10-9 shows a right shoulder with the arthroscope in the posterolateral portal, inflow in the posterior portal, and positioning needles in the anterolateral and anteromedial corners of the acromion.

Next, a lateral working portal is created using a point 0.1 cm posterior and 2 to 3 cm lateral to the anterolateral corner of the acromion (Fig. 10-10; also see Fig. 10-3). If necessary, a trochar may be used to eliminate fluid extravasation and facilitate insertion for surgical instruments. Initial visualization in the subacromial space will often be quite poor, especially in cases of true impingement tendinitis caused by chronic fibrosis of the subacromial space. Patience is necessary at this point in the procedure to achieve adequate excision of the subacromial bursa as necessary for visualization of the undersurface of the acromion. Although triangulation is vital, it is helpful to have an appreciation of depth by placing a similar scope or arthroplasty instrument on the skin and comparing this with the depth of the surgical instrument. Eventually, with the cutting surface toward the acromion, enough soft tissue will be resected to provide a space to visualize a field in which to work. A large, 5.5 mm, full-radius synovial resector is ideal for this part of the procedure.

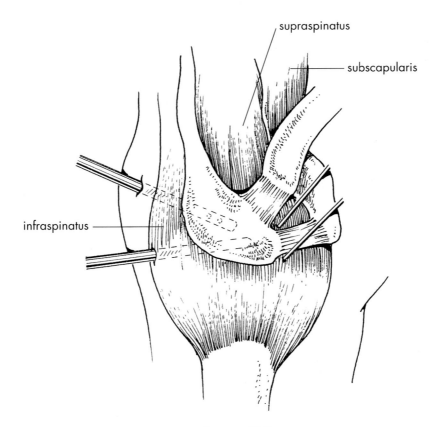

FIGURE 10-9

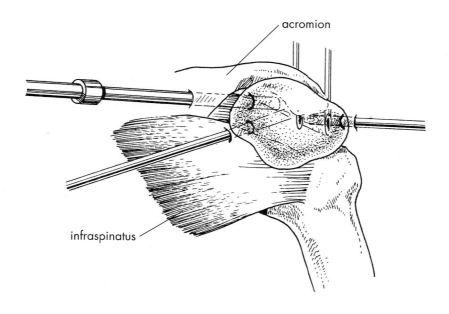

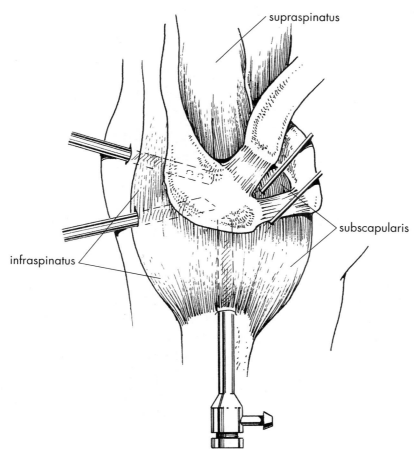

FIGURE 10-10

In those cases of profound thickening of the coracoacromial ligament and bursal tissue beneath the acromion, it is helpful to first release this tissue with electrocautery (Fig. 10-11). The shaver system will then have a better "foothold" from which to work. Fig. 10-11 shows this technique looking at the subacromial space from behind.

Anatomical landmarks that should be visualized before bony resection include the coracoacromial ligament anteriorly, the anterolateral corner of the acromion, the acromioclavicular fat pad immediately beneath the joint medially, and the medial and the anterior margin of the acromion. When these landmarks are visualized and outlined, adequate resection of the bursa has been accomplished and acromial decompression may be started.

Various sizes and shapes of burrs are commercially available, ranging from 4.5 mm to 6.5 mm in oval, cylindrical, or pear-shaped designs. Surgeons must be comfortable with the aggressiveness of the given instrumentation and, therefore, should use the smaller, less aggressive burrs early in the learning curve, until they are technically proficient. We typically use a 5.5 mm, pear-shaped burr, entering from the lateral portal. We begin our decompression at the anterolateral corner of the acromion (Fig. 10-12).

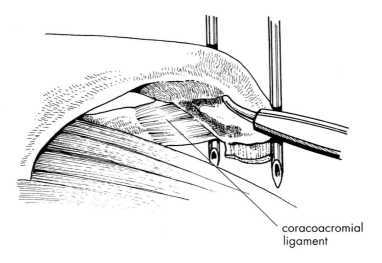

coracoacromial
ligament

FIGURE 10-11

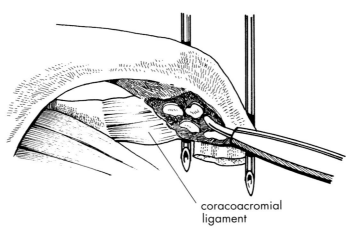

coracoacromial
ligament

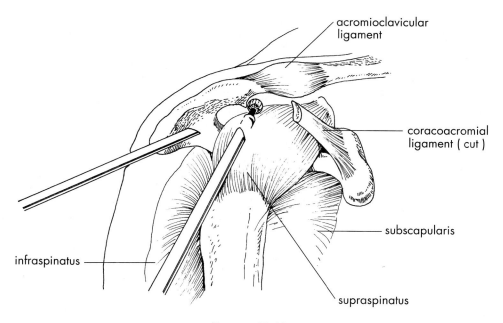

acromioclavicular
ligament

coracoacromial
ligament (cut)

subscapularis

infraspinatus

supraspinatus

FIGURE 10-12

In cases of a marked hook to the acromion or in individuals with a prominent lateral margin, this area must be decompressed first to gain access to the more medial aspect of the acromion during the remaining decompression. Working lateral to medial (Fig. 10-13, *A*) and anterior to posterior, the surgeon resects sequential layers of the acromion. Some surgeons initially prefer to fully decompress the anterior 0.5 cm of the acromion from medial to lateral and then complete the remainder of the acromioplasty in a gradual fashion posteriorly. During the process of decompression, the coracoacromial ligament is also released from the anteroinferior acromion (Fig. 10-13, *B*).

Hemostasis during shoulder arthroscopy is extremely important for proper visualization, especially in subacromial work. There are four methods to help maintain hemostasis: electrocautery, hypotensive anesthesia, pump inflow, and epinephrine. Electrocautery is very effective, even in a saline medium, and allows immediate control of specific bleeders. Hypotensive anesthesia is best applied with a general anesthetic, a systolic pressure of 90 mm Hg being ideal. This method is much better achieved under general anesthesia, but it is very difficult to achieve under scalene block anesthesia, especially when the patient is in the sitting position. Pump inflow allows periodic increases in the inflow pressure to exceed the mean arterial pressure and to control bleeding. Epinephrine may be mixed with bags of inflow, creating a 1/300,000 concentration. In our setting, a combination of mild hypotensive and regional scalene anesthesia, pump inflow, and electrocautery has been effective.

In most instances, an adequate decompression has been achieved when the superior or superficial cortex of the acromion has been encountered. A gentle transition from anterior to posterior should also be accomplished, providing appropriate decompression. Viewed from the lateral aspect, Fig. 10-14 shows an adequate decompression, with the transition of the decompression being at the apex of the concavity of the acromion, thus converting a Type III acromion to a Type I. By placing the camera laterally, the burr can be brought in posteriorly to complete the decompression. Some surgeons perform most of the decompression with the burr in the posterior portal. Viewed from the undersurface of the acromion, Fig. 10-13, *B* shows a smooth, uniform decompression from lateral to medial and anterior to posterior. A guide to decompression may be the width of the burr. In this case, a 5.5-mm burr is used and our desired resection is 1.5 to 2 cm from anterior to posterior. Three widths of the burr and a smooth decompression should confirm an adequate resection.

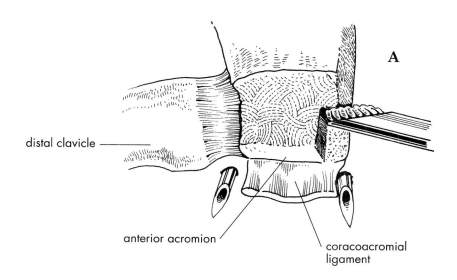

distal clavicle

anterior acromion

coracoacromial
ligament

A

FIGURE 10-13

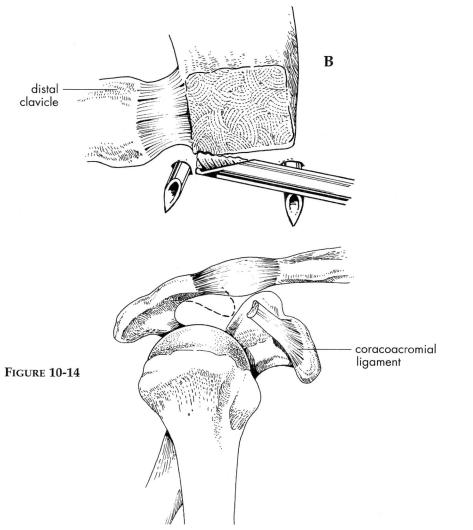

distal
clavicle

B

coracoacromial
ligament

FIGURE 10-14

In the initial stages of performing an acromioplasty or if there is any concern about the adequacy of decompression, a finger may be inserted through an enlarged lateral portal and a rasp used to smooth any residual areas of prominence. With a finger in the lateral portal, the rotator cuff can be palpated to detect any tears.

Once an adequate decompression has been accomplished, the surgeon should inspect the rotator cuff and debride any associated bursal tears. Full thickness rotator cuff tears may then be approached by a formal arthrotomy, lateral miniarthrotomy, or both.

Closure

At the completion of the procedure, all instrumentation is removed, portals are closed with subcuticular stitches, and a local long-acting anesthetic is injected into the subacromial space for postoperative pain relief. A drain may be used and removed before discharge from the outpatient facility. The patient is placed in a sling and swathe for comfort and taken to the recovery room.

POSTOPERATIVE CARE (SEE CHAPTER 11)

All patients are placed in a cryotherapy shoulder cuff to minimize postoperative edema and pain. If an interscalene block has been used, only an oral analgesic is given for pain control. If, however, a general anesthetic has been used, the patient may be discharged with a patient-controlled analgesia machine to allow intermittent parenteral analgesic dosage. Patients may be hospitalized overnight. Patients are warned about drainage from the portals during the following 24 to 48 hours and are instructed in appropriate dressing changes. Passive motion is started immediately; in the case of regional interscalene blocks, this may be in the recovery room.

A formal physical therapy program is taught to the patient preoperatively and reinforced in the recovery room. Initially, passive exercises are undertaken for a few days, proceeding to active exercises as soon as pain and motion allow, in approximately 4 to 5 days. At the time of the first office visit 1 week later, motion is checked and modifications in the program are made. Resistive exercises are added at 3 to 4 weeks. A return to manual labor might be anticipated at 3 months.

Arthroscopic Bankart Repair (Suture Technique - Caspari)
GENERAL CONSIDERATIONS

Arthroscopic repairs for unstable shoulders involve one of three distinct techniques: a transglenoid suture, an anterior glenoid tack device, or anterior suture anchors combined with sutures. It is now possible to tie the sutures down as would be performed in an open Bankart repair. The transglenoid suture technique, first described by Drs. Caspari and Morgan, has proved to be reproducible by some surgeons, but not all. A modification of this technique described by Dr. Wolf uses anterior glenoid suture anchors, thus avoiding the need for transglenoid drilling. All of these procedures demand meticulous preparation of the anterior glenoid, proper suture placement, and tensioning of the soft tissues for success. Because of the small size of sutures used to repair the glenolabral complex and because of the less than ideal security of the repair, most surgeons immobilize these patients in an adducted, internally rotated position for 3 or 4 weeks postoperatively. As these procedures technically become better and we are able to approach the security of an open Bankart repair, the advantage of early mobilization will parallel our open procedures.

Indications

These techniques are applicable to individuals with well-defined Bankart lesions. Patients with only capsular laxity may be addressed arthroscopically; however, open capsulorrhaphy remains the standard treatment of choice for those patients.

Expectations

As in open procedures, the expectation in this technique is a stable shoulder. Some might argue that because of the less invasive technique, patient morbidity is reduced and, thus, the technique may be performed on an outpatient basis or an overnight stay. Failure rates are reportedly higher with the arthroscopic technique, especially in contact athletes. Current rehabilitation is slower because patients are immobilized for 3 to 4 weeks. Stiffness may, therefore, be less predictable. However, most patients will note a return to their preinjury functional status with a preserved range of motion.

SURGICAL TECHNIQUE

Positioning

Positioning for an instability procedure in the lateral position is aided by the use of a dual traction system (see Figs. 2-7 and 2-8). The arm is placed in 15° of abduction with slight axial traction. A second traction line is placed about the upper arm and directed cephalad to help pull the humeral head laterally away from the glenoid. Finally, the body is rolled posteriorly 30° to bring the glenoid face parallel with the floor, making instrumentation of the glenoid rim easier (see Fig. 2-5, C).

The sitting position for shoulder stabilization, in our experience, is slightly more difficult but can be used (see Fig. 2-2). This position requires someone to apply traction to the arm to distract the humeral head.

Procedure

Basic portals are used initially employed with diagnostic arthroscopy carried out by a standard posterior portal. The superior, or supraspinatus, portal may be established for inflow if the sensor is not on the scope (see Fig. 10-6). If the sensor is on the scope, the superior portal is unnecessary. An anterior working portal is established in the subscapularis triangle by an inside out technique (see Fig. 10-4). It is helpful to use a second anterosuperior portal for visualization, instrumentation, or both to have a better approach to the anterior labral complex (Fig. 10-15; also see Fig. 10-5). Having identified the Bankart lesion, free tissue is debrided, a 4 mm burr is inserted, and the anterior rim of the glenoid is decorticated (Fig. 10-16). With the Caspari technique, because of the suture punch size, a larger cannula is necessary, which is inserted in the anterior working portal. Sutures are placed in sequential fashion, beginning inferiorly at the anterior band of the inferior glenohumeral ligament and labrum and working superiorly up to the middle glenohumeral ligament and labrum (Fig. 10-17).

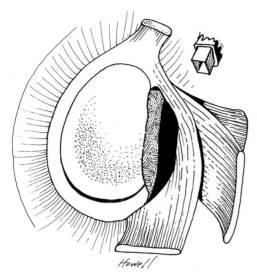

FIGURE 10-15

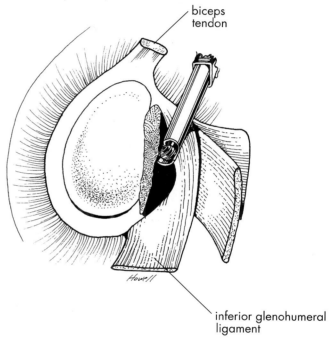

biceps
tendon

inferior glenohumeral
ligament

FIGURE 10-16

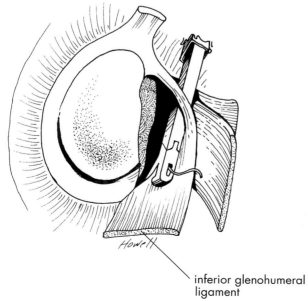

inferior glenohumeral
ligament

FIGURE 10-17

Several technical tips may help to avoid a rather steep learning curve for this procedure. First, we have found that an 0-size monofilament absorbable suture is optimal relative to the size of the suture punch. Second, after having grasped the tissue, feed the suture so that the end is just past the wheel on the handle. Open the tine of the grasper, rotate, and slowly begin to withdraw the suture punch. As you withdraw the punch with the tine open, the remaining suture should pass easily down the shaft of the suture punch and both ends will be free as the punch is removed from the cannula. After all sutures are in place, tension is applied to ensure good soft tissue purchase (Fig. 10-18).

The next step is drilling of the glenoid neck to pass the sutures, a step that represents a potentially large area for error. It is important that two planes be correctly maintained throughout the drilling process, both coronal and sagittal. As Fig. 10-19 shows, not only does the drill bit have to be directed deep and medial relative to the articular surface of the glenoid, but it must also be directed caudally, aiming toward the mid portion of the scapula. Ideally, one would like to exit on the skin slightly medial to the midpoint of the scapular spine and 5 to 6 cm inferior to it. This will incorporate the appropriate degree of inferior and medial displacement for the drill bit (Fig. 10-20). The orientation of this tunnel is crucial. By viewing from behind (Fig. 10-21, *A*), from above (Fig. 10-21, *B*), and from the side (Fig. 10-21, *C*), one can better understand the direction the drill is to take. Although close to some branches of the suprascapular nerve, this exit point for the drill should avoid injuring the main trunk because of its lateral and inferior position (Fig. 10-22).

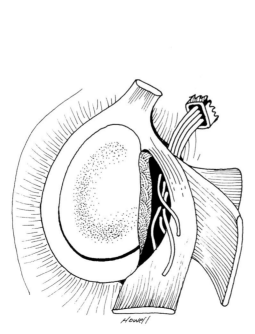

FIGURE 10-18

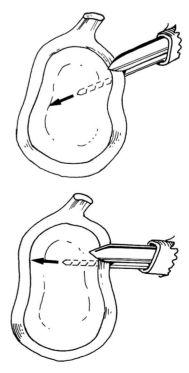

FIGURE 10-19

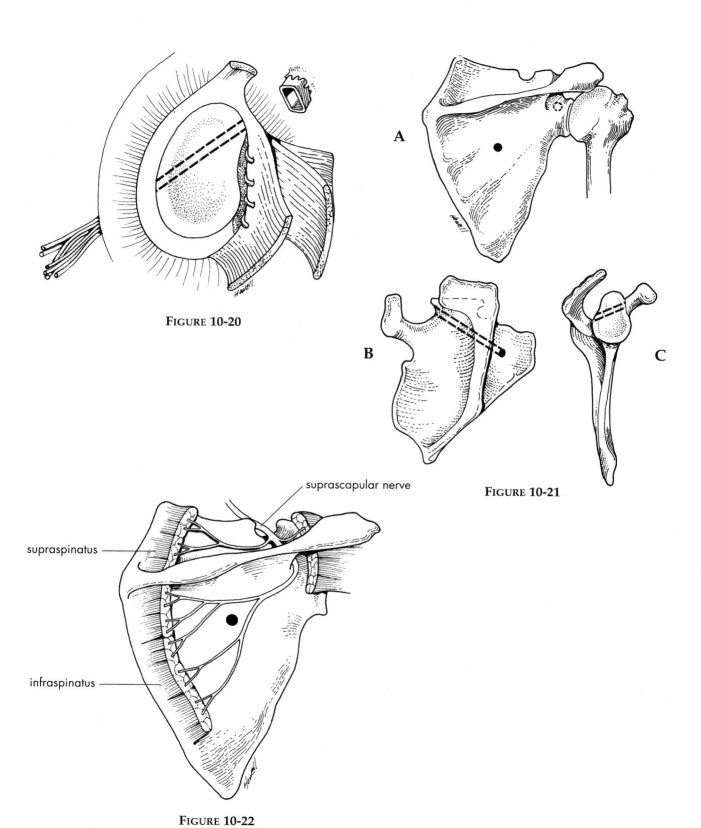

FIGURE 10-20

A

B

C

FIGURE 10-21

suprascapular nerve

supraspinatus

infraspinatus

FIGURE 10-22

Once through both cortices, a small, 2-cm incision is made at the drill's exit point in the skin posteriorly and the sutures are brought through the neck of the glenoid and the posterior soft tissues with the drill bit. The sutures are split into two bundles and a large-eyed French cutting needle is used to pass one bundle through, incorporating the thick posterior fascia (Fig. 10-23). Traction is released, the arm is brought down into an adducted, internally rotated position, and the sutures are tied. Some surgeons advocate dissecting down to the posterior glenoid neck and then tying these sutures, thus minimizing interposed soft tissue posteriorly. This may provide better tensioning of the repair.

With the Morgan technique, large bore needles with an eye in the end can be placed through the anterior portal to secure the anterior soft tissue complex. The sharp point can then be drilled through the glenoid neck, exiting in the middle of the infraspinatus fossa. A suture is placed on the end of this. The pin can be pulled through with one suture coming out the back and the remaining suture left at the front (Fig. 10-24, A). This procedure can be duplicated through the same cannula with another needle, grabbing tissue just a few millimeters adjacent to the previous suture and again drilling through, coming out at roughly the same exit point in the infraspinatus fossa. The suture at the front can be placed in the eye of this needle and pulled through, allowing a mattress effect to secure the anterior glenoid labrum and capsule to the glenoid neck (Fig. 10-24, B). These are then tied over the infraspinatus fascia. The procedure is otherwise much the same as the Caspari technique. Several mattress sutures can be placed if desired.

Closure

All the portals are closed with a subcuticular stitch, and a light compressive dressing is applied. The patient is placed in a sling and taken to the recovery room.

POSTOPERATIVE CARE (SEE CHAPTER 11)

The patient is allowed to remove the sling for hygienic reasons. At all other times, the sling must remain in place with the arm internally rotated and adducted. This is maintained for the first 2 weeks, at which time gentle pendulum exercises are added. Between 3 and 4 weeks, passive elevation and external rotation are started. At 5 weeks, active forward elevation, external rotation, and internal rotation are performed, carefully monitoring external rotation, aiming for near full motion by 12 weeks. Resisted exercises for rotational and scapular strengthening begin at 6 weeks.

By 2 months, 75% of motion should have returned and isokinetic strengthening exercises may be added for endurance. Also, gentle throwing exercises may be started with an anticipated resumption of full throwing motion at 4 months. Contact sports are avoided for a minimum of 4 to 5 months.

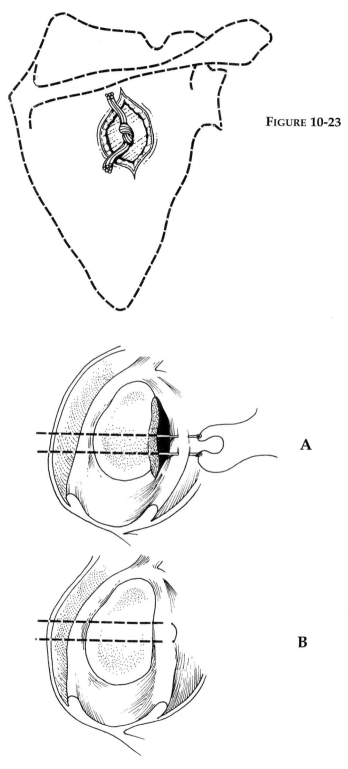

A

B

FIGURE 10-24

Arthroscopic Bankart Repair (Glenoid Tack Fixation)
GENERAL CONSIDERATIONS

Significant developmental strides have been made in glenoid fixation devices. Beginning with metal staples and screws, later evolving into suture anchors with arthroscopic knot-tying devices, the field has come full circle, back to the original concept of a tack; the difference now is that there are resorbable devices with varying half lives. The application of these devices remains technically demanding and avoids the need for multiple sutures and transglenoid drilling. There is the risk, however, as with their metallic predecessors, of loosening, joint irritation, foreign body reaction, and questionable fixation.

Indications

This system is best used in the patient with a large, well-defined Bankart lesion and no associated capsular laxity. At this time, relative contraindications would be poor quality soft tissue and multidirectional instability.

SURGICAL TECHNIQUE
Positioning

Positioning for an instability procedure in the lateral position is aided by the use of a dual traction system (see Figs. 2-7 and 2-8). The arm is placed in 15° of abduction with slight axial traction. A second traction line is placed about the upper arm and directed cephalad to help pull the humeral head laterally away from the glenoid. Finally, the body is rolled posteriorly 30° to bring the glenoid face parallel with the floor, making instrumentation of the glenoid rim easier (see Fig. 2-6).

The sitting position to stabilize the shoulder, in our experience, is slightly more difficult but can be used (see Fig. 2-2). This position requires someone to apply traction to the arm to distract the humeral head.

Procedure

The posterior portal is used for viewing, and a thorough inspection of the glenohumeral joint precedes any operative treatment for the instability. Initially, the anterior portal is created along with an anterosuperior portal. The anterosuperior portal is created with a cannula to allow preparation of the anterior glenoid. The anterior portal is subsequently created from inside out, the anterosuperior portal from outside in. Either a rasp or small burr is used to prepare the glenoid surface for subsequent reattachment of the glenolabral complex (Fig. 10-25; also see Fig. 10-16). Using the same anterosuperior portal, a grasper is inserted to hold the middle and inferior glenohumeral ligaments and is drawn superiorly to both confirm mobility of this complex and to assess the amount of superior displacement that will be possible at the time of tack fixation (Fig. 10-26). Once the anterior glenoid is adequately prepared, a second working portal is created just superior to the tendinous border of the subscapularis. A portal may be established into the substance of the upper subscapularis if desired. The more medial the portal, the more effective the right angle into the angled anterior glenoid neck (always staying lateral to the coracoid).

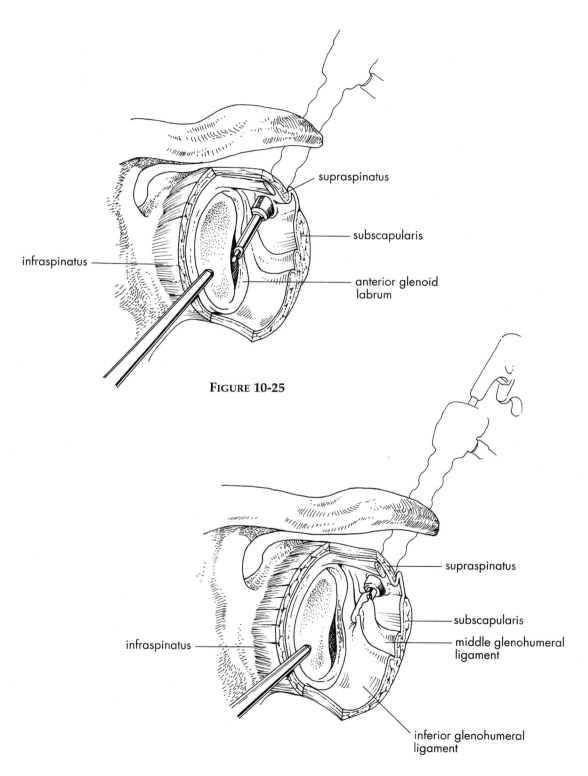

FIGURE 10-25

FIGURE 10-26

A cannulated drill bit with guide wire is inserted through this portal and while the capsulolabral complex is drawn superiorly, the soft tissues are speared and the guide wire is placed against the anterior glenoid rim (Fig. 10-27).

Viewed from above with a tangential cut through the glenoid, we can see how the soft tissue is pinned to the anterior rim with the guide wire (Fig. 10-28). The drill is then inserted to the depth of at least one marking on the drill guide, which will ensure adequate depth for subsequent tack placement (Fig. 10-29). The guide wire is tapped to lock it into place, and the cannulated drill is gently removed. A tack is inserted over the drill guide, followed by the tack impactor (Figs. 10-30 and 10-31).

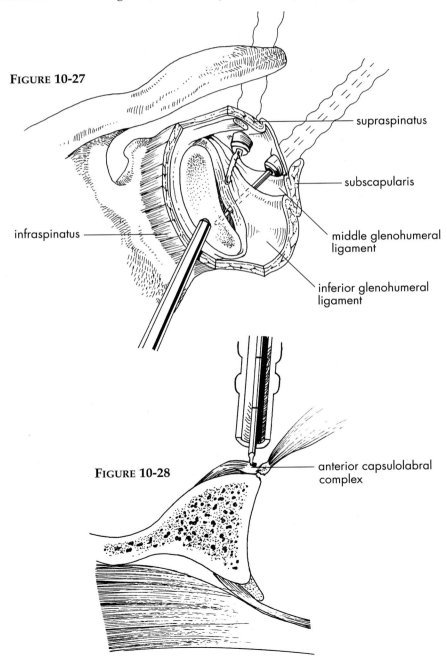

FIGURE 10-27

supraspinatus

subscapularis

middle glenohumeral ligament

inferior glenohumeral ligament

infraspinatus

FIGURE 10-28

anterior capsulolabral complex

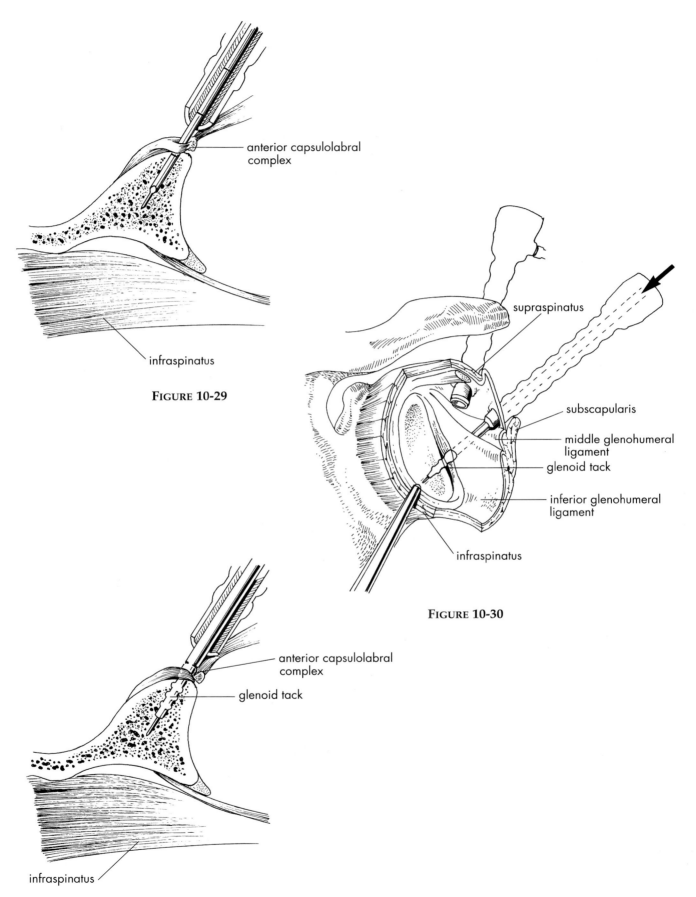

anterior capsulolabral complex

infraspinatus

FIGURE 10-29

supraspinatus

subscapularis

middle glenohumeral ligament

glenoid tack

inferior glenohumeral ligament

infraspinatus

FIGURE 10-30

anterior capsulolabral complex

glenoid tack

infraspinatus

FIGURE 10-31

An additional tack may be placed superiorly as needed (Fig. 10-32). It is difficult to position a tack inferiorly. It is helpful to grasp the head of the tack through the anterior portal to test its security before accepting the situation as being secure.

POSTOPERATIVE CARE (SEE CHAPTER 11)

The patient is allowed to remove of the sling for hygienic reasons. At all other times the sling must remain in place with the arm internally rotated and adducted. This placement is maintained for the initial 2 weeks, at which time gentle pendulum exercises are added. Between 3 and 4 weeks, passive elevation and external rotation are started. At 5 weeks, active forward elevation, external rotation, and internal rotation are performed, carefully monitoring external rotation, aiming for near full motion by 12 weeks. Resisted rotational and scapular exercises are started at 6 weeks.

By 2 months, 75% of motion should have returned and isokinetic strengthening exercises may be added for endurance. Gentle throwing exercises may be started, with an anticipated resumption of full throwing motion at 4 months. Contact sports are avoided for a minimum of 4 to 5 months.

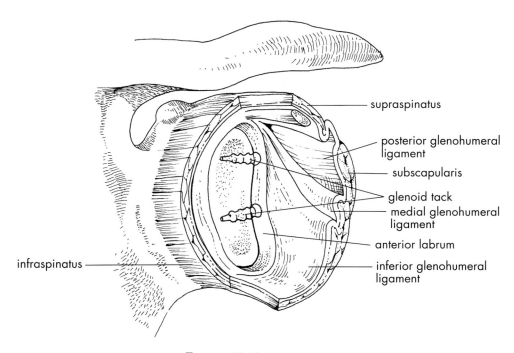

FIGURE 10-32

Arthroscopic Bankart Repair (Metallic Suture Anchor Fixation)
GENERAL CONSIDERATIONS

Anterior reconstructions using suture fixation have the advantage of multiple point fixation and minimal tissue trauma. Remember that Caspari's technique is only one point of fixation. The disadvantage of the Caspari system is the requisite transglenoid drilling and knot placement posteriorly over fascia. Not only is there a risk associated with drill placement, but there is also the risk of posterior soft tissue compression and suprascapular nerve injury. In response to this, Dr. Wolf developed an arthroscopic technique for anterior repairs using the existing Mitec suture anchor system. Other systems, such as the Revo (Linvatic) and absorbable anchors, are available or will be soon. The advantage of this technique is that it most closely reapproximates the techniques used in open repairs. All fixation is anterior, and there is an anatomical repair of the Bankart lesion. Unlike the tack system, there is no risk of a prominent or poorly secured fixation device. An arthroscopic Bankart repair, from the front, is our preferred method of fixation, allowing an early aggressive rehabilitation program and approaching outcomes that are comparable to an open Bankart repair.

Indications

The indications for this technique are similar to those of the previous techniques— a well-defined Bankart lesion with reasonable soft tissue. One advantage of this system is that some capsular tightening can be accomplished by advancement of the inferior capsulolabral complex and the inferior glenohumeral ligament.

Expectations

The majority of these patients will notice a successful result with elimination of instability symptoms and a return to functional activities, approaching the results of an open Bankart repair. Unfortunately, it is a technical challenge, compromising success to some degree.

SURGICAL TECHNIQUE
Positioning

Positioning for an instability procedure in the lateral position is aided by the use of a dual traction system (see Figs. 2-7 and 2-8). The arm is placed in 15° of abduction with slight axial traction. A second traction line is placed about the upper arm and directed cephalad to help pull the humeral head laterally away from the glenoid (see Figs. 2-7 and 2-8). Finally, the body is rolled posteriorly 30° to bring the glenoid face parallel with the floor, making instrumentation of the glenoid rim easier (see Fig. 2-6).

The sitting position to stabilize the shoulder, in our experience, is slightly more difficult but can be used (see Fig. 2-2). This position requires someone to apply traction to the arm to distract the humeral head.

Procedure

Having completed an examination under anesthesia and a glenohumeral inspection with the arthroscope, three portals are established—both anterior (see Fig. 10-4) and anterosuperior (see Fig. 10-5) working portals and a posterior portal for viewing (see Fig. 10-1). Preparation of the glenoid neck is performed with soft tissue and burring instruments to prepare a good bed for ultimate bony fixation (see Figs. 10-16 and 10-25). With the Bankart lesion well defined and its degree of mobility determined with a grasping instrument, insertion holes for the anchors are all predrilled with the appropriate drill for the set (Fig. 10-33). Drilling is best performed with the camera positioned in the posterior portal. Visualization of the anterior glenoid is best performed with the camera in the anterosuperior portal.

The passage of sutures begins inferiorly at the anterior band of the inferior glenohumeral ligament complex, using a suture passer to place a 0 monofilament suture (Fig. 10-34). The suture is then grasped and pulled back through the cannula (Fig. 10-35). The inner limb of the suture is passed through the Mitec (Fig. 10-36), which is fully inserted under direct visualization into the previously drilled hole (Fig. 10-37).

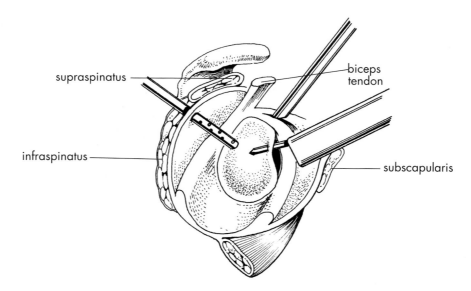

supraspinatus

biceps tendon

infraspinatus

subscapularis

FIGURE 10-33

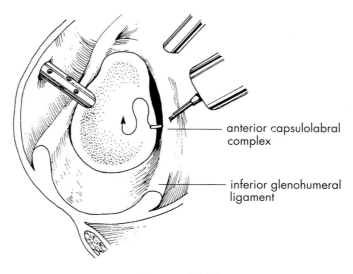

anterior capsulolabral complex

inferior glenohumeral ligament

FIGURE 10-34

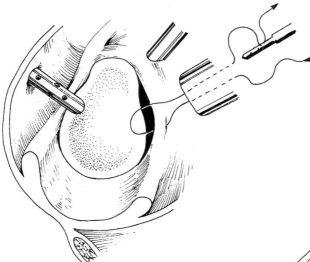

FIGURE 10-35

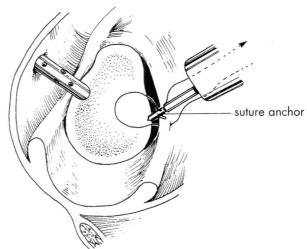

suture anchor

FIGURE 10-36

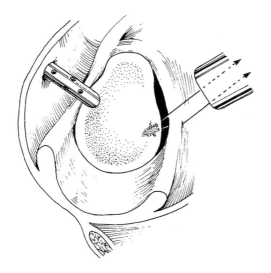

FIGURE 10-37

The two free ends of the suture that pass through the Mitec and through the capsulolabral tissue are then knotted, using a slip knot (Fig. 10-38). With a knot pusher, they are tightened against the labral construct (Fig. 10-39). This process is repeated two or three times with the result being a stable repair with apposition of soft tissue to anterior glenoid bone (Fig. 10-40).

Closure

Closure is routine with removal of instrumentation, subcuticular stitches for the portals, and application of a sling and swathe.

POSTOPERATIVE CARE (SEE CHAPTER 11)

The patient is allowed to remove the sling for hygienic reasons. At all other times, the sling must remain in place with the arm internally rotated and adducted. This position is maintained for the first 2 weeks, at which time gentle pendulum exercises are added. Between 3 and 4 weeks, passive elevation and external rotation are started. At 5 weeks, active forward elevation, external rotation, and internal rotation are performed (carefully monitoring external rotation) aiming for near full motion by 12 weeks.

By 2 months, 75% of motion should have returned and isokinetic strengthening exercises may be added for endurance. Gentle throwing exercises may be started, with an anticipated resumption of full throwing motion at 4 months. Contact sports are avoided for a minimum of 4 to 5 months.

In the future, absorbable anchors will become available and these will be a great advantage compared with nonabsorbable materials. Dr. Snyder has developed a suture shuttle that allows a movement of sutures through soft tissue in an organized fashion.

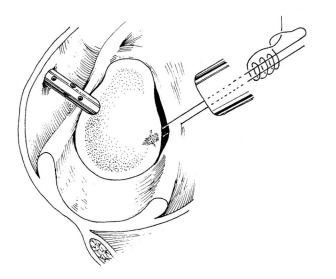

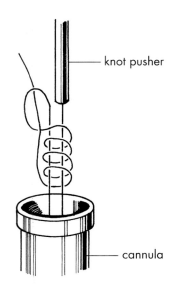

knot pusher

cannula

FIGURE 10-38

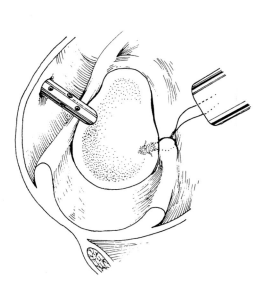

FIGURE 10-39

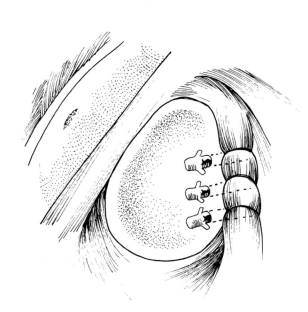

FIGURE 10-40

ARTHROSCOPIC BANKART REPAIR USING THE SUTURE SHUTTLE TECHNIQUE

The variation using the suture shuttle varies slightly from the previously described technique. Using the suture shuttle technique, drill holes are placed in the anterior glenoid and an anchor is positioned in these drill holes. With this device, either a modified punch or a Curly-Q shuttle passer is inserted through the glenoid labrum (Fig. 10-41). One arm of the shuttle is exited through one of the anterior portals, and a free limb of the suture from the previously positioned anchor is inserted into the suture shuttle device. The shuttle is then pulled from the glenoid to the opposite cannula to incorporate the anterior glenoid and labrum. Both arms of this suture arrangement are brought out one portal and appropriately tied into position to create a Bankart type of repair, as in the open repair. This is repeated three times, again hoping to achieve a secure Bankart repair.

This technique allows a normal postoperative program, as in an open Bankart repair, consisting of early range of motion exercises, passively limiting external rotation to approximately 30° for 2 weeks. At 2 weeks, active range of motion exercises are started, limiting external rotation to approximately 45° until 4 weeks. The sling is removed between 2 and 3 weeks. At 4 weeks, active exercises with terminal stretching are continued, progressing slowly to full external rotation at 4 to 12 weeks. Resisted exercises are started at 4 weeks.

At 3 months, the patient is allowed to return to sporting activities, although contact sports are delayed until 4 months. If throwing activities are involved, normal aggressive overhead motion is not allowed for 6 to 12 months.

FIXATION OF SLAP LESION

We prefer to fix a SLAP (Superior Labral Anterior Posterior) lesion using either the tack system (Figs. 10-25 through 10-32) or the suture system (Figs. 10-33 through 10-39).

Two anterior portals are established with visualization from the posterior portal. The tack or suture anchor can be inserted through the anterior superior portal. For a posterior SLAP fixation, the tack or anchor must be inserted from a position slightly posterior to the anterior lateral corner of the acromion (Fig. 10-42).

Arthroscopic Acromioclavicular Arthroplasty (Distal Clavicle Resection)
GENERAL CONSIDERATIONS

As the use of the arthroscope in the shoulder increases, so has the variety of its applications. Recently, several individuals have begun reporting successful results with arthroscopic acromioclavicular arthroplasties for arthritis and post-traumatic painful joints. Distal clavicle resection, if done arthroscopically, is more easily accomplished following an arthroscopic subacromial decompression. In these cases, the acromial facet of the joint has been resected, exposing the distal clavicle for subsequent resection. In contrast, an isolated distal clavicle resection is somewhat more tedious. It requires various sizes of arthroscopes and instrumentation. However, it can be very successful and is a reproducible technique. There are two approaches to resection of the outer clavicle. The first technique is in conjunction with an anterior acromioplasty. After completing the acromioplasty, the burr is brought medially to the acromioclavicular joint, and the inferior half of the distal clavicle is excised. The superior half is resected, using an additional anterior portal.

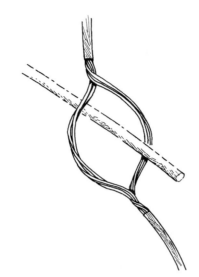

FIGURE 10-41

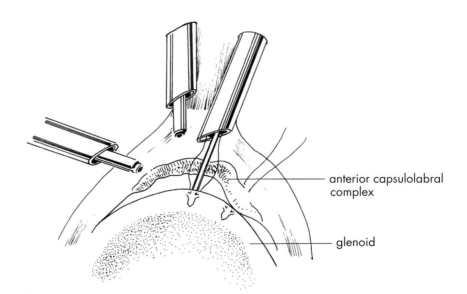

anterior capsulolabral
complex

glenoid

FIGURE 10-42

The second technique is a more direct approach to the acromioclavicular joint alone. This technique uses small instruments initially from superior anterior and superior posterior to the joint. Larger instruments are then used to complete the resection.

Indications

The ideal patient is one with isolated acromioclavicular arthritis, minimal acromial changes, and at least some preservation of the joint space. Coexistent impingement or rotator cuff tear are better addressed with an ASD and clavicular resection or an open cuff repair, respectively.

Expectations

Over 90% of these patients will note pain relief and return to normal function. The postoperative morbidity is minimal. This technique may be performed on an outpatient basis or overnight stay.

SURGICAL TECHNIQUE
Positioning

Like most arthroscopic procedures, this technique places the patient in a lateral decubitus position (see Fig. 2-4). A sitting position (see Fig. 2-2) may be used, depending upon the surgeon's preference. The "beach chair" position may also be used (see Fig. 2-1).

Procedure

An examination under anesthesia and a glenohumeral inspection are performed before any acromioclavicular joint work, noting any cuff pathology, subacromial changes, and the like. If the clavicular resection is to be done in combination with an ASD, the acromioplasty is performed in standard fashion. Viewing is from the posterior portal, while resection is from the lateral portal. It is imperative that the decompression be adequate to provide reasonable visualization of the articular surface of the clavicle. The key to this is an adequate resection of the acromial facet of the acromioclavicular joint. With the acromioplasty complete (see the section on ASD), the burr is brought more medially over to the inferior half of the distal clavicle. Resection begins posteriorly and works anteriorly (Fig. 10-43). Looking at this from the subacromial space up toward the undersurface of the acromion, note that the acromioplasty is complete and that the burr is now being brought over to the lateral aspect of the distal clavicle, resecting the inferior half of the joint. This resection from the lateral portal continues until the burr abuts on the undersurface of the acromion. Digital downward pressure of the clavicle may bring the residual portion of the distal clavicle into view for additional resection. An additional anterior working portal is used immediately anterior to the acromioclavicular joint. The burr is introduced through this portal, and the residual superior portion of the distal clavicle is then resected (Fig. 10-44). The arthroscope may be moved to the lateral portal, thereby giving a direct view of the clavicle. In most cases, with a 25° or 30° arthroscope, visualization of the acromioclavicular joint is adequate from the posterior or posterolateral portals.

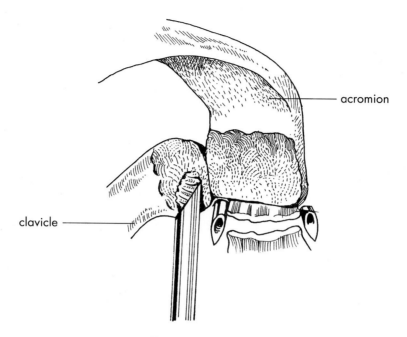

FIGURE 10-43

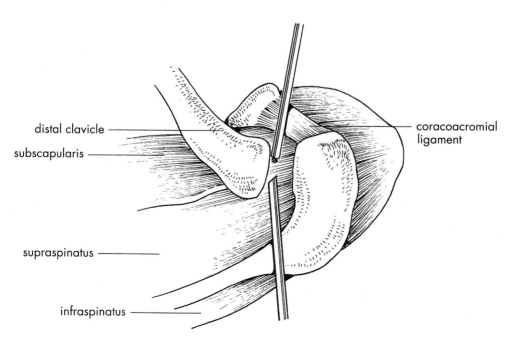

FIGURE 10-44

In those individuals with preservation of the joint space, such as patients with idiopathic osteolysis or weightlifter's shoulder, a direct acromioclavicular arthroplasty may be done arthroscopically. This procedure is performed by introducing the arthroscope immediately posterior to the acromioclavicular joint, using the superior portal but directing the cannula anteriorly. To start, a small 2.7 arthroscope may be necessary to initiate the procedure because of the limited space available. In many individuals with idiopathic osteolysis, however, the joint space will be adequate to use a 4 mm arthroscope. An anterior working portal is created and, if necessary, a superior inflow portal. Viewing posteriorly and working anteriorly, the anterior one half or two thirds of the distal clavicle is resected to a depth of approximately 1 to 1.5 cm (Fig. 10-45). The instrumentation is now switched, using switching sticks, so that our viewing portal will be anterior and our working portal posterior (Fig. 10-46). The residual posterior rim is resected in this fashion so that we have a uniform decompression of 1 to 1.5 cm. If necessary, it is possible to resect the acromial side of the acromioclavicular joint to further decompress this area.

Closure

All instrumentation is removed, the joint is injected with a long-acting analgesic, and the portals are closed with subcuticular stitches and Steristrips. The patient is placed in a sling.

POSTOPERATIVE CARE (SEE CHAPTER 11)

The patient is allowed to start on active and passive range of motion exercises immediately. Passive motion is carried out for the first few days, progressing to active motion at 4 to 5 days, and resisted motion at 2 to 3 weeks. When range of motion is full, isokinetic strengthening is added and most patients return to work, athletic endeavors, or both at approximately 8 weeks.

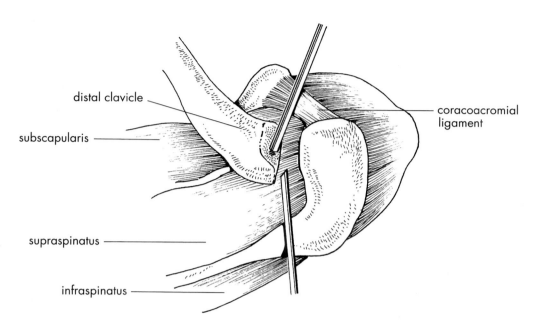

FIGURE 10-45

distal clavicle

subscapularis

supraspinatus

infraspinatus

coracoacromial
ligament

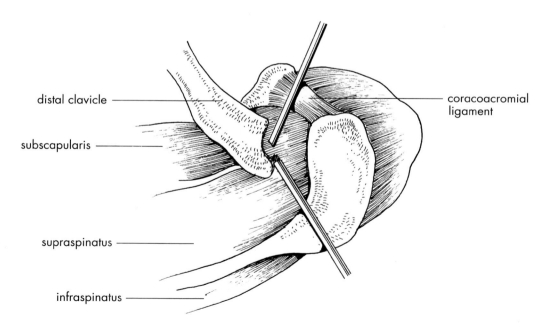

FIGURE 10-46

distal clavicle

subscapularis

supraspinatus

infraspinatus

coracoacromial
ligament

Rehabilitation

11

Many factors must be considered in an approach to rehabilitation of the operated shoulder. The usual program progresses through the following three phases:

PHASE I - passive or assisted exercises to gain motion
PHASE II - active exercises with ongoing terminal stretching exercises
PHASE III - resisted exercises with ongoing active and terminal stretching program (that is, Phase II)

The rate of progression of this program depends on several factors:

1. Pain
2. Approach to managing the deltoid
3. Underlying reconstructive procedure
4. Demands of the patient
5. Aggressiveness and nature of the surgeon

The critical issue in rehabilitation relates to the timing of when active exercises are started, allowing the muscles to work on their own. In most operative procedures about the shoulder, the active (Phase II) program can be started as soon as pain and motion allow, often within days or weeks, depending on the magnitude of the reconstruction, the amount of pain, and the progression of the postoperative Phase I program. There are obvious situations when tissues must be protected until healing occurs before active motion can be started. These situations include rotator cuff reconstructions, fracture fixations, or other procedures in which tissue planes have been violated, such as in a large deltoid takedown. Even in these circumstances, Phase I can often be started immediately, even if a brace is used, until active motion is allowed. Active motion (Phase II) is frequently delayed for 6 to 8 weeks, depending on the time to healing of the violated tissues. Resisted exercises can then be implemented several weeks after Phase II.

When progressing from the Phase I to the Phase II program following large reconstructions, the patient must often return to the supine position because of significant weakness. Often, patients can actively elevate their arms in the supine position, but not in the upright position, where the lever arm is much more influential. As strength improves and pain permits, the patient can progress to the sitting and upright positions. This progression can occur with the patient initially supine, then with the upper torso inclined 30°, 60°, and finally 90°. A lawn chair is ideal for such a program.

If immobilization is required for tissue healing, such as in multidirectional instability, arthrodesis, certain fracture patterns, or large reconstructions, a spica cast, a commercial orthotic splint, or some form of abduction pillow may be used. The position required for each of these procedures is determined by the surgery and the surgeon. In circumstances such as nonunion surgery, inferior capsular shifts, or other large reconstructions, complete immobilization may be required until tissue healing occurs. In other circumstances, exercises above the level of the immobilized position can be instituted, thus allowing the rehabilitation program to progress.

The rehabilitation program requires meticulous instruction and careful monitoring by both surgeon and physiotherapist. A close relationship with clear communication between therapist and surgeon is essential to success. The patient must to understand the timing of the various phases, the expectations along the way, and the eventual expected outcome. For example, in rotator cuff reconstructions, it is important to tell patients that it will probably be 6 months before they will be able to elevate their arm on their own above the horizontal with comfort and confidence.

It is appropriate to teach the patient the program, have the patient assume responsibility for performing the exercises, and have appropriate follow-up visits when the program needs changing. This instruction will avoid confusion and simplify the process as much as possible. In the early days and weeks following an operative procedure, frequent sessions are required, perhaps 5 times per day, 10 to 15 minutes each for each session, with an assigned number of repetitions for each exercise. The number of times per day can be diminished to three and then one, depending on timing, progress, operative procedure, and surgeon's preference. It is important to remind patients that once they are discharged from physiotherapy, stretching and strengthening once per day are worthwhile.

Phase I—Passive or Assisted Exercises

The initial motions to be gained in as relaxed and pain-free manner as possible are elevation and external and internal rotation. It is helpful initially to exercise in the supine position, depending on pain and procedure, progressing to upright, as pain and progress permit. The power for an assisted or passive program is from the opposite normal extremity or, in the presence of bilateral disease, may be from such aids as pulleys and sticks. The motion is taken to the point of pain, stressed a little farther, held for the count of three or four, and returned to the resting position. As long as pain does not linger, the appropriate amount of tissue stretching is occurring. The goal is obviously to gain degrees each time and each day. Forward elevation is usually done with the opposite arm powering the operated arm upward (Fig. 11-1). Some patients prefer some traction on the arm with elevation, others prefer a bent elbow position. Supine (Fig. 11-2) and upright (Fig. 11-3) external rotation, with the arm at the side and the elbow fairly snug to the body, is aided with a stick. Internal rotation is performed with a stick to achieve extension the first few times and then reaching behind the back with the opposite extremity to pull the arm and hand up the back (Fig. 11-4). Initially, this is done 4 or 5 times per day, with perhaps 10 repetitions of each exercise. Pendulum exercises as a warm-up can be added after 1 or 2 days and are used as a warm-up at the beginning of all programs (Fig. 11-5). In most surgical procedures, Phase I can be started the day of surgery, particularly if an interscalene block is used for postoperative pain control. After a few days, most exercises can be done in the upright position.

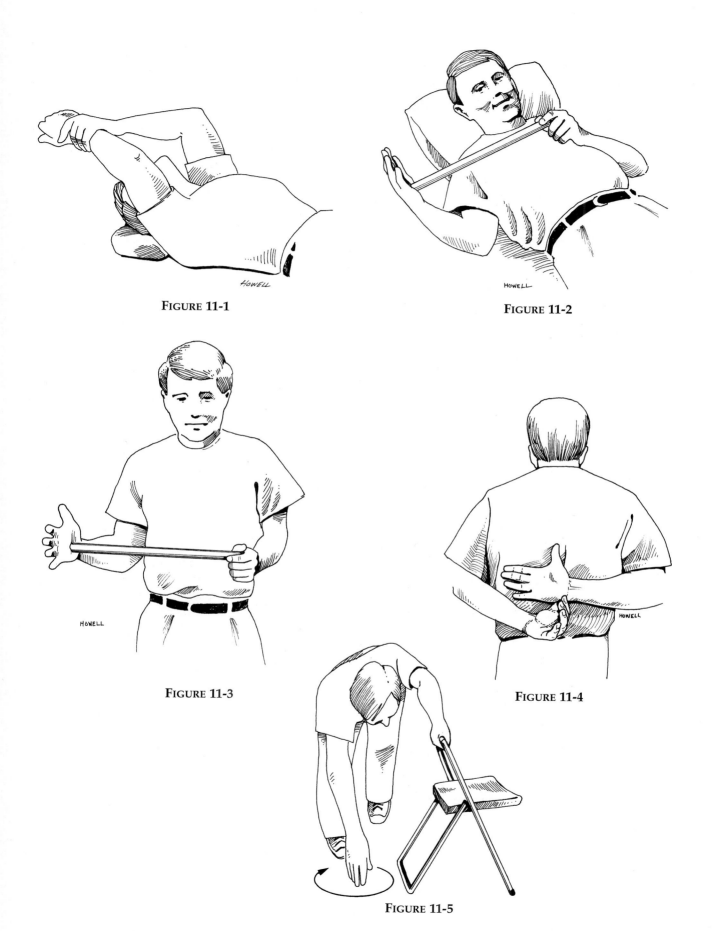

FIGURE 11-1

FIGURE 11-2

FIGURE 11-3

FIGURE 11-4

FIGURE 11-5

The Phase I program continues until motion progresses satisfactorily, pain diminishes, and the underlying reconstruction is secure. At that time, Phase II (active motion) is started.

Phase II—Active Exercises with Terminal Stretch

When passive motion has progressed satisfactorily and pain has diminished, Phase II (the active phase of the program) can be started. With rotator cuff tears, fracture fixation, or large deltoid reconstructions, this phase is delayed until tissue healing has occurred. With large reconstructions, especially if the shoulder is still painful and weak, the patient should return to the supine position, particularly for elevation. This position effectively shortens the lever arm. As strength improves, the patient can progress to the upright position.

The motions to gain are the same as in the passive program—forward elevation, external rotation with the arm at the side, and internal rotation. In the supine or upright position, the patient elevates the arm forward as far as strength will allow. The patient then grasps the wrist of the operated arm with the normal arm (as in the passive program) and pushes the operated arm toward full elevation. At this point, the normal arm releases the operated arm. The operated arm is held in a fully elevated position and then slowly brought down in an eccentric fashion to the patient's side.

External rotation is performed with the arm at the side and the patient actively externally rotating as far as possible. Using either a stick or the normal arm, the patient stretches the operated arm terminally to full external rotation, the stick or normal arm is removed, and the operated arm is held in full external rotation and then brought slowly back across the abdomen to rest.

Internal rotation is performed actively using the normal arm and terminal stretching. Pendulum exercises are continued as a warm-up. This phase of the program continues for a variable time, depending on the patient and the pathology, but usually lasts for 4 weeks. During this phase, terminal stretching is usually an ongoing part of the program. The frequency of Phase II exercises depends on the pathology and the patient's schedule, but is usually three times per day. The number of repetitions varies, but is usually between 10 and 20 for each exercise.

Phase III—Resisted Exercises with Ongoing Phase II

Phase II continues as the patient progresses to Phase III. Phase III, or resisted exercises to strengthen the muscles, begins when appropriate active motion has been achieved, pain is under control, and the arm is strong enough to undergo resisted exercises. Postoperatively, the muscles to be strengthened are the external and internal rotators and the forward elevators. This strengthening can be performed in many ways but is usually best performed with some form of resistance rubber exercisers such as a Sport Cord or Thera-Band. These exercises can be performed while sitting or standing.

External rotation can be performed (Fig. 11-6) with the arm at the side and the elbow snug to the body. This positioning allows concentric strengthening of the infraspinatus and, upon return, allows eccentric strengthening of the infraspinatus. This maneuver can be reversed with the patient facing the opposite direction with resisted internal rotation and the arm slowly brought back to neutral with external rotation (Fig. 11-7).

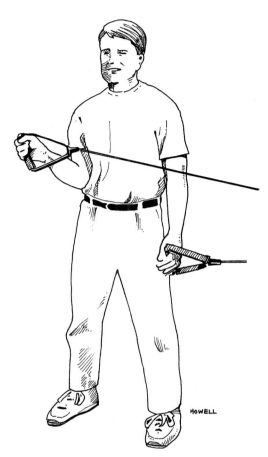

FIGURE 11-6

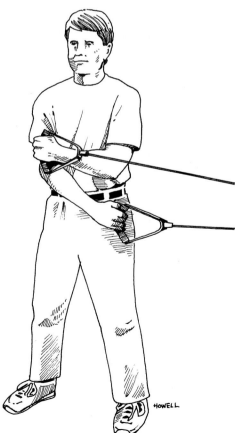

FIGURE 11-7

This exercise is concentric for the internal rotators, such as the subscapularis, and eccentric for the internal rotators as the arm is brought back to the neutral position. The rubber exerciser can be put in the door or on a door handle. In the relaxed position, the arm can be slowly thrust forward in a punching maneuver and brought back slowly to strengthen the anterior deltoid, both concentrically and eccentrically (Fig. 11-8). Because there is often some degree of deltoid violation surgically and sometimes even subtle neurological involvement, it is important to work on the anterior deltoid for elevation.

During this phase of resisted exercises, Phase II continues with active exercises and terminal stretching to ensure maximum motion. This program is continued for many months until normal or near-normal strength and motion have been obtained.

Because more aggressive stretching is desired for the terminal degrees of elevation and for external and internal rotation, special techniques can be used, such as hanging from the door for forward elevation (Fig. 11-9) and pushing the operated arm out while the normal arm is supported in a door jamb for external rotation (Fig. 11-10). The number of times the Phase III program is implemented depends upon the patient's schedule, the surgery performed, and the progress of the patient's rehabilitation. It should be at least twice per day and between 10 and 20 repetitions for each exercise.

As the patient progresses and the shoulder nears complete rehabilitation, the patient needs only to perform a simple stretching and strengthening program for a few minutes each day to maintain the motion and strength of the shoulder.

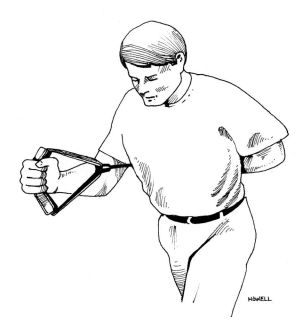

FIGURE 11-8

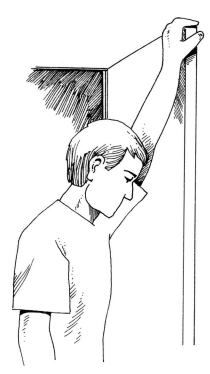

FIGURE 11-9

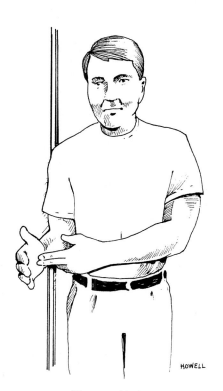

FIGURE 11-10

Special Considerations in the Athelete

Sometimes in select patients, particularly competitive athletes such as throwers, a more sophisticated program is used. The phases progress similarly, although perhaps slower, and the emphasis eventually becomes focused on selective strengthening in a functional manner. For example, in a thrower or swimmer, part of the emphasis would be on eccentric subscapularis and infraspinatus rotational strengthening and scapulothoracic strengthening. We prefer a form of resistive rubber tubing, such as a Sport Cord exerciser for external and internal strengthening at neutral and 45° elevation in the scapular plane (Fig. 11-11). Strengthening is done at 90° of elevation only in the terminal phases and only if the patient is asymptomatic.

In addition to anterior deltoid strengthening, focus is directed to the scapular musculatures to stabilize the scapula as it rotates on the chest wall (Fig. 11-12). Seated rows are performed for the rhomboids and serratus anterior muscles. Upright shrugs are performed for the trapezius (Fig. 11-13). These exercises are directed toward scapular efficiency.

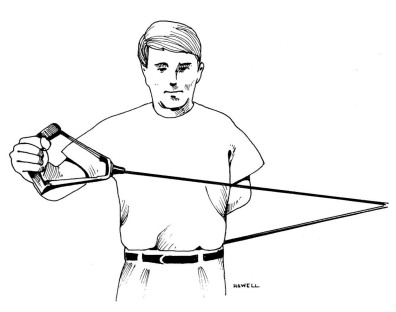

FIGURE 11-11

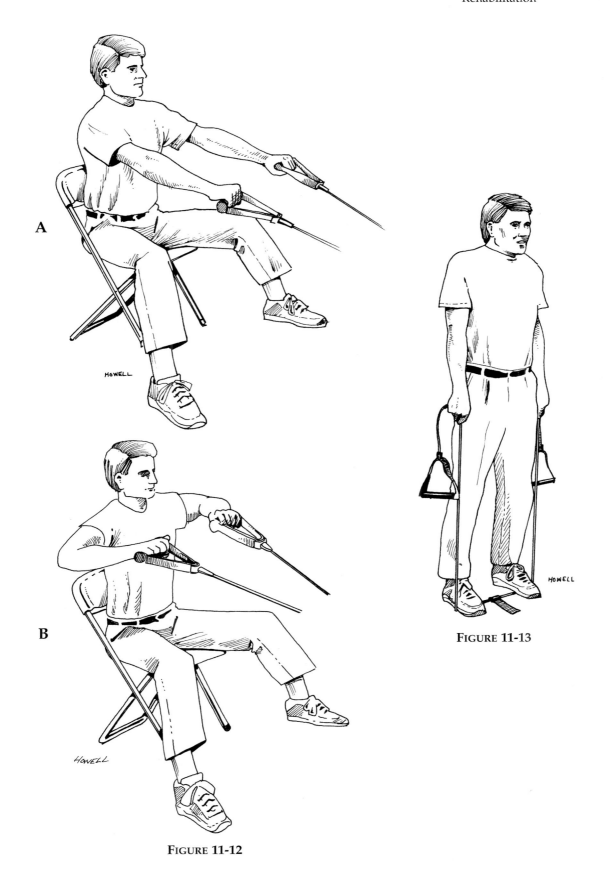

A

HOWELL

B

HOWELL

FIGURE 11-12

HOWELL

FIGURE 11-13

Closely supervised use of isokinetic machines may be considered in the high-profile athletic population with caution. We are concerned about the unsupervised use of such machinery. Many athletes prefer a free-weight training program, which should be carefully monitored (Fig. 11-14). Postoperatively, we discourage certain heavy overhead weight training such as bench and military presses, especially in the wide-arm position. These exercises put excessive stress on the anterior capsule and are particularly dangerous after stabilizing procedures. Fig. 11-14 shows a method of strengthening the anterior deltoid following major reconstructions, by progressing from supine, to inclined, and finally to upright positions. Often, following major reconstructions when the deltoid is weak, such a program allows gradual upright elevation.

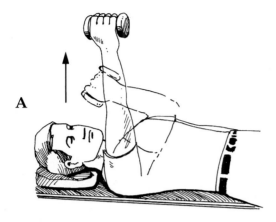

A

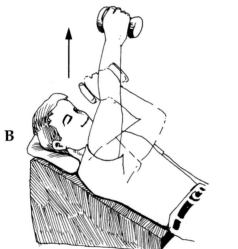

B

FIGURE 11-14

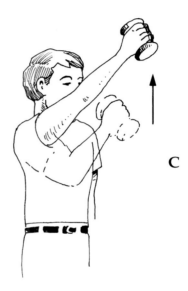

C

Index

Z